Includes An Epigenetic Modifier Program

OBESITY GENES

and
THEIR EPIGENETIC MODIFIERS

James D. Baird, PhD

Author of *Happiness Genes*
An Amazon Kindle best seller for biology

OBESITY GENES

Disclaimer: This book and its programs are not designed to replace medical or psychiatric treatments for a serious health condition. Please seek professional help if you have questions about your physical or psychological health

A production of
HWL. Inc

934 Cherry Hills Lane, Naperville IL 60563
Copyright © 2012 James D. Baird, PhD
All rights reserved.
ISBN: 1477420142
ISBN 13: 9781477420140

TABLE OF CONTENTS

Introduction vii

Chapter 1 –What this book can do for you 1
1. The problem restated 1
2. Why you bought this book 2
3. Overweight, obesity and hypertension are hazardous to
   your health 4
4. How obesity and hypertension are defined 5
5. How does American rate in world health 8
6. Why this book is unique, and credible 11
7. The Obesity Gene Diet [OGD] 11
8. Healthy Longevity of HALL people 14
9. The Obesity Genes bottom line 16
10. The promises of the book 17
11. What do you have to do? 18

Chapter 2 – The Genesis of our obesity epidemic 19
Introduction 20
1. Our 'obesity genes' under control 20
2. Our fat programming 21
3. Our sweetness programming 22
4. Our instinct for inactivity 23
5. The nature of our obesity genes 23
6. Genes out of sync 26
7. Our changing eating patterns 27
8. Our biological systems for bodyweight outmatched 34
9. Examples of encouraging our obesity genes 36
10. Epic changes in our environment in the latter
    part of the 20th century 38
    a. Family environment 38
    b. Inactivity 40
    c. Food Processing 41

   d. Levels of Development... 44
   e. Psychological 47
   f. Food Consumer 48

CHAPTER 3- Why weight loss programs can be weight gain programs **53**
  1. Background... 53
  2. Popular trends in current diets.................................... 54
  3. The yo-yo effect 56
  4. Weight loss drugs are not the answer.......................... 56
  5. about carbohydrates.. 59
  6. Major types of diets... 61
  7. Why popular diets can't work?.................................... 70
  8. Why the EMP does work 71

CHAPTER FOUR − The Worlds healthiest and longest lived [HALL] peoples...**73**
  The Elder Okinawans,.. 73
  Traditional rural Chinese.. 78
  Traditional Mediterranean Countries 83

CHAPTER 5 − The EMP eating program **91**
  1. The bottom line... 91
  2. Avoid these foods 93
  3. The skinny on fats... 94
  4. EMP food choices at a glance...................................... 96
  5. Serving sizes.. 97
  6. Recommended food groups.. 97
  7. Preparing vegetables 97
  8. Helpful Hints 99
  9. Eat multiple meals 100
 10. Summary xxx

CHAPTER 6 − How the EMP behavioral program makes it work **103**

1. The goals of the program.. 104
2. The biology of the Program.. 105
3. The EMP 6 month outline 107
4. The first month plan-4 acts 109
5. What is mindfulness?... 109
6. Following your breath 112
7. Act 1-Mindful eating... 114
8. Act 2-Eat from food group 115
9. Act 3 -Consume less calories 117
10. Act 4-Burn 100 calories a day − 118
11. Activity calories table.. 120
12. Daily Acts Journal 121
13. Month two −Changing eating habits............................... 122
14. Understanding EMP Self Hypnosis 124
    a. What is self-hypnosis?.. 124
    b. Your conscious and subconscious mind...................... 125
    c. Changing eating habits and reasons for eating 127
    d. Install posthypnotic eating suggestions..................... 127
    e. Components of the EMP plan 128
15. Self-Hypnosis induction script 134

CHAPTER 7-Exercise, physical activity and weight control..... 143
    1. How physical Activity helps control weight..................... 143
    2. The Health Benefits of physical activity 145
    3. The right amount of physical activity............................. 146
    4. Moderate-intensity activity 147
    5. Aerobic activity.. 148
    6. Stretching and Muscle Strengthening Exercises............. 149
    7. Tips to a safe and successful physical activity program ... 151

Appendix A − Recommended Food Groups 155
Appendix B − Recommended foods by nutrient density,
              Glycemic index and fiber.................................. 157
Appendix C − Typical Menus 165
Appendix D − Sources and Citations −................................. 173

INTRODUCTION

Overview

The problem

The exponential rise of obesity in America has quickly come to rival heart disease and cancer as the number one health problem facing our society today. Recent reports show that obesity in the United States increased by 61% in just the past 10 years. It's now thought that between 25 and 30% of all adults in the US are obese. When considering overweight individuals, almost 60% of adults fall into the categories of overweight/obese, and the trend is escalating. Multiple studies are linking obesity to reduced quality of life in addition to such devastating diseases as; cancer, coronary artery disease, diabetes, and Alzheimer's. It's no surprise that more people than ever are searching for a way to lose weight permanently and become fit.

Unfortunately, while most diets can result in initial weigh losses, they fail to maintain the weight loss, and it all too soon returns. In a recent analysis, Dr Dansinger, and colleagues of the Tufts New England Medical Center looked at results from 46 weight loss diet studies totaling nearly 12,000 participants. Writing in the *Annals of Internal Medicine,* they reported that the average weight loss was just 6% and that most dieters regained all the weight they lost within five years. No diet significantly bettered that average.

Verifying these results, The National Institutes of Health states that the majority of diets fail in the first year, and over 90% fail within 5 years. These findings come as no surprise, since it is common knowledge that 'diets don't work'. In desperation, the public keeps trying each new diet variation, hoping that this one will work for them. But their hope is based on false assumptions, and their efforts predestined to failure.

The basic reason for this is that, it's not the diet that fails, but rather the dieter fails to maintain the diet. The simple biological fact of diets is that, if we reduce calorie intake and/or burn more calories, we will lose weight, and if we continue to do this, we will weigh less, no matter what the diet. But while the strategy of losing weight is simple, the execution is not. The reality if that; reducing calorie intake, changing food preferences, and burning more calories are complex issues that are linked with our prehistoric instincts, and our modern culture.

The cause of the problem

So the question becomes, is there a realistic way for the dieter to maintain a healthy diet, or is we doomed to get fatter and more obese? This book answers this question, by first explaining the major causes why most are unable to maintain their diet.

- **Genetics** - a powerful set of 'obesity' genes inherited from the ancient days when humans lived a feast-or-famine existence. To lose weight and keep it off, we must acknowledge the power of our genetic heritage, modify our obesity genes and find healthy ways to work *with* our natural cravings for sweets, fats and calories.

- **Insufficient physical activity** - the technological advances of our modern world has substantially reduced the need for physical activity, accepting our genetic instinct to reduce burning calories.

- **Unhealthy eating habits** – We are creatures of habit, and consequently attempting to change to less tasty and healthier foods without changing our eating habits is destined to failure.

Over the past 35 years, researchers studying populations predisposed to obesity such as the Pima Indians have discovered a set of genetic traits that work against most people who are trying to adopt healthier habits while surrounded by modern temptations of inexpensive, high caloric foods. Numerous studies published in journals such as *The Journal of Internal Medicine* and the *American Journal of Clinical Nutrition* have identified a set of 10 to 20 individual genes–collectively called "the thrifty genotype"–that encode our food preferences and make us crave fatty, sugary foods. As soon as the body senses fewer calories are coming in, these genes direct the body to turn up hunger sensations and cravings for high calorie foods. It's no wonder that such genetic programming eventually erodes even the strongest self-motivation, causing the dieter to give in to the temptations that lead to weight gain. On top of our genetic predisposition to obesity, for the past 50 years Americans have been living in a society that has increasingly encouraged us to cater to our "fat" genes. Fast food restaurants, packaged foods, and vending machines let us access food in an instant. We now live in a hyper caloric society where our genetic predisposition for high calorie foods can be fully satiated 24 hours a day, 7 days a week.

Healthy diets

Studies conducted by nutrition researcher Ancel Keys and others during the 1950s and 1960s and recently expanded upon by Harvard's Walter Willett, M.D. show that a diet rich in vegetables, nuts, fish, olives, plant fats, and whole grains provides the perfect ingredients for both weight loss and longevity. Keys' landmark Seven Countries Study, which examined the dietary patterns and health of people in seven different countries, found that the world's longest lived people in Mediterranean areas such as the Greek island of Crete stay slender by consuming most of their calories from vegetarian foods and by physical activity each day. Other major nutritional studies, such as Campbell's Cornell China study and Wilcox's 25-year study of Okinawa reveal similar results; the foundation of a healthy weight and a long life is regular physical activity, a diet rich in natural plant foods, and healthy eating habits.

Adopting healthy diets

Since what people prefer to eat is a learned habit, we can learn to change our eating habits and food preference. One way of doing that is to relocate to a healthier culture

And, as is common, adopting the indigenous foods. However, this is obviously not realistic for most people. So, the issue is, how do you change your food preferences from the typical American diet based on animal products and excessive calories, to one based on plant foods and less calories, and enjoy the transition? When most people learn they must eat more vegetables and cut back on animal products, there is an instant thought of 'no way'. It seems totally unrealistic.

But it can only not be done, but accomplished with minimum effort, by following the step by step process of the EMP program. The Obesity Genes Diet [OGD]acknowledges that it is futile to fight our 'obesity' genes and meets their demands for fat, sweets and calories with healthy fats [olive oil, canola], healthy sweets [fruits] and calories [unlimited vegetables and fruits]. The Obesity Genes Diet [OGD] is a tasty blend of the diets of the worlds healthiest and longest living peoples [HALL], the Mediterranean, Asian, and Okinawa cultures. While this is a good initial start, without a change of eating habits, the OGD would soon be fall by the wayside, as other diets do.

Changing eating habits

To work permanently, you're eating habits must be changed so that you prefer to eat the OGD. The epigenetic modifiers presented in this book, are proven to be able to modify behavior, and eating preferences. For many years, psychologists have taught self-hypnosis techniques to help patients do everything from change their lifestyle habits to overcome pain syndromes. One recent study of

60 overweight women published in the *Journal of Consulting and Clinical Psychology* found that self-hypnosis combined with a healthful diet resulted in twice as much weight loss as dietary changes alone. Easy-to-learn self-hypnosis techniques have been specially designed in script and/or CD and can be learned in as little as 5 to 10 minutes a day. While you are learning how to change your eating habits, other EMP modalities, such as mindfulness, will help convert the unhealthy habits in your subconscious, to make the transition pleasant. Another important cornerstone of the EMP program is physical activity. Research done on people who have lost significant weight and kept the weight off for a year or more shows that physical activity is necessary for any successful weight loss program. Readers will be taught how to slowly increase the amount of time they spend with physical activity each day, choosing from an array of options to prevent boredom and increase motivation. Included in the EMP self-hypnosis intervention, are inductions for habits that will make physical activity desirable and automatic.

How long does it take?

The goal of the Obesity Genes program is to lose an average of 1 lb. /week until you reach your desired weight and then stabilize. Those who are more overweight, may well lose more, but gradual and consistent is the key to long term maintenance. A significant change of eating habits is reasonable within 4 months, assuming a time/effort investment of 15 minutes/day performing epigenetic exercises for the first few months. Those who put forth more practice reap quicker rewards. However, in no case, should you increase your effort to the point that the program becomes uncomfortable, as this will discourage your continued effort. As time goes by and the practices become automatic, they will be ingrained into your life style and conscious effort will be unnecessary.

The Program

The Program is divided into three phases.

- During phase 1, readers learn food guidelines and follow them during one of their daily meals. During their other meals and snacks, they may eat whatever they desire. The Obesity Genes Diet is rich in fiber, vegetable protein, and plant foods. The food guidelines include ample fats from nuts and olive oil and sweet flavors from fruit to satisfy hunger and innate cravings. Simultaneously, readers will practice mindful eating during one meal a day, using the mindful eating mind state to increase their awareness of what and how much they are eating, eat more slowly, savor their food. During one meal, they learn the eating tips that will allow them to eat 5-10% less calories than normal. During this phase, readers also adopt a physical activity goal of burning 100 extra calories a day.

- Phase 2 is focused on changing eating habits by behavioral self-hypnosis after the foundational work of Phase 1 is completed. As epigenetic interventions are practiced, eating healthy requires less and less effort, as perceptions epigenetically modify our obesity genes. Readers also expand what they learned in phase 1—practicing the food guidelines during two daily meals and eating mindfully at all meals. They increase their exercise goal to burning 200 additional calories a day. During this second phase, readers learn by how to change their eating habits by specially designed self-hypnosis and imaging programs.

- Phase 3 concerns reinforcement of your new eating habits, and a thorough understanding of healthy eating habits. Continuous practice of mindfulness will keep you aware of what you are eating and why, so that you don't slip back into unhealthy habits. Living mindfully 'living in the moment' is not only an effective way to avoid subconscious eating, but also one of the best epigenetic interventions to reduce fear, worry, and stress.

CHAPTER ONE

What this book can do for you

1. The problem restated
2. Why you bought this book
3. Overweight, obesity and hypertension are unhealthy
4. How obesity and hypertension are defined
5. How does American rate in world health
6. Why this book is unique, and credible
7. The Obesity Gene Diet [OGD]
8. Healthy Longevity of HALL people
9. The Obesity Genes bottom line
10. The promises of the book
11. What do you have to do?

1. The problem restated

As discussed in the introduction we are under siege from an escalating health crisis that has the potential of being the most disastrous health crisis the U.S. has ever experienced. The signs of the problem and its consequences are everywhere.

- 50 million adults in the U.S. have high blood pressure.
- Two−thirds of all Americans are overweight or obese.
- The reduced quality of life of the overweight and obese
- Obesity at youth equals a loss of 20 years of life

1

- Losing weight can prevent one out of every 6 deaths from cancer
- Our children now account for one third of new Type 2 diabetes cases
- The cost of overweight and obese to the US economy is difficult to overestimate?
- There are no practical and acceptable proven programs for effective treatment
- 95% of diets fail within five years
- Since the cause is genetic, this is a worldwide pandemic.
- Obesity attributes to at least 300,000 deaths a year.
- If the trend continues, obesity will double in 20 years
- Obesity causes huge increases in heart disease, stroke, cancer and other diseases
- American is the most significant leader in the obesity trend.

AND WORSE – FROM A NATIONAL PERSPECTIVE, THERE IS PRESENTLY NO WORKABLE WAY IN SIGHT TO STOP THIS RUNAWAY TREND

2. Why you bought this book

While the national and world view is chilling enough - the reason you bought this book is to improve your quality of life and solve this health threat for yourself. And after you have done that, hopefully you will want to help others by spreading your story. There are hundreds of books, theories, concepts, opinions; etc. selling different ways to lose weight, but the cold fact of reality is that virtual none will produce long term weight loss let alone healthy weight loss. That's not just opinion, it's simply a fact documented by our National Institutes of Health. So why this book? Perhaps you recognized that this program is unique and since the diets you tried don't work, maybe this will. Or maybe the concept rings true that the cause is genetic and that it's not your fault. You have been caught between your obesity genes and an encouraging environment, a situation where your will power working sporadically, is no match for genes working 24/7. But you are probably skeptical, and rightly so, self-help books have a poor reputation for changing lives. But that's just the point, they don't work for the same reason diets don't work, because they don't provide a plan to change our genetic habits. That food preference and quantity is a habit is simple to observe and we see this frequently. If you were born in China, you probably would love bean sprouts, but if you relocated to the U.S. it wouldn't be very long before you preferred the local fare.

But if you are just interested in weight loss, why not just burn more calories than you eat? The reason is that you are not going to be happy if you are hungry all the time, and you will not be able to develop a habit that keeps you in pain. Not to mention the damage to your health. Then how does the problem get solved by changing your food preferences and eating habits? Because it is a proven fact that there are peoples that live longer, are slimmer and less disabled then Americans. For convenience we call them world's healthiest and longest lived peoples, or HALL peoples. They enjoy a health significantly better than the US, in spite of our outstanding resources and medical technology. The important question is how to adopt the healthy food preferences and lifestyles of the HALL people in our environment of Western food and the ever present consumer food media?

Short of relocating to the land of the HALL peoples, the quickest and most practical way is to change your genetic eating habits. Our epigenetic program is a step by step self-administered program designed to convert your habits so that you prefer the diets and lifestyles of the HALL people. These programs can be learned by following the specially designed scripts daily until your new eating habits become established. The practices are designed for all types of people, regardless of experience or personality. Previous experience at getting out of your unconscious mind is helpful, but not necessary.

3. Being Overweight, Obese, or Hypertensive is Unhealthy

As previously mentioned, over two thirds of all Americans are overweight, and about one-third are more than overweight – they are actually obese, an unhealthy condition that sets us up for major illnesses and shortened healthy life-spans. The prevalence of obesity in the United States has doubled in the last 20 years with studies showing that 31% of adult Americans are obese, according to the U.S. Department of Health and Human Services (HHS). "The problem keeps getting worse and has profound health implications" says HHS Secretary Tommy Thompson. Americans have a soaring rate of hypertension according to two recent reports released by the U. S. government.

Hypertension, also known as high blood pressure, is an especially serious medical condition that causes early death and disability. Fifty million adults in the United States – including more than one of every two adults over the age of 60 – have high blood pressure, according to the National Center for Health Statistics. Even scarier is that data from the National Heart, Lung and Blood Institute's landmark Framingham Heart Study suggests that middle-aged and elderly U.S. citizens face a 90% risk of developing hypertension during their remaining years

Recent estimates attribute more than 300,000 deaths each year in the U.S. to obesity. According to the American Institute for Cancer Research (AICR), over 100 research studies consistently link obesity to post-menopausal breast cancer, colon cancer, endometrial cancer, prostate, and kidney cancer. If you are overweight, you are also more likely to develop serious health problems such as hypertension, heart disease, stroke, Type 2 diabetes, gallbladder disease, and gout (joint pain caused by excess uric acid).[1] Furthermore, in women obesity commonly causes infertility problems, irregular menstrual flow, and urinary incontinence. The good news is that losing as little as 10% of your current excess weight will help to lower your risk of developing certain obesity-

---

1

related diseases including hypertension. Recent studies indicate that a modest loss of 5% to 10% of body weight can lower blood pressure and reduce your risk of developing diabetes, heart disease, stroke, and even cancer, the leading diseases that cause premature death and disability.

"Epidemiological data suggest that if we could lower the average systolic blood pressure among Americans by 5 mmHg, we'd see a 14% drop in deaths from stroke, a 9% drop in heart disease deaths, and a seven percent drop in overall mortality," says Dr. Paul

Whelton, senior vice president for health sciences for Tulane University Health Sciences Center and co-chair of the National High Blood Pressure Education Program supported by the National Heart, Lung, and Blood Institute [NHLBI]. According to the NHLBI press statement, "Proven behavioral changes can lower one's blood pressure and reduce the risk of a cardiovascular disease . . . In one study overweight participants with normal BP levels significantly lowered their systolic BP by losing fewer than eight pounds."

In the largest study of its kind, researchers with American Cancer Society followed almost one million cancer free men and women for 16 years the study showed that people who were overweight had a higher risk of dying from cancer. Researchers estimated that overweight and obesity could account for 14 percent of all deaths from cancer in men and 20 percent in women. The obese with a Body Mass Index [described below] of at least 40 had death rates that were over 50% higher. [New England Journal of Medicine, April 24, 2003]

4. How obesity and hypertension are defined

Body fat, is necessary and desirable, we all need a certain amount of body fat for stored energy, heat insulation, shock absorption and other functions. It's the amount and location of the body fat that presents the health problems. Overweight is an excess of body weight compared to set standards. It may come from muscle, bone, fat and or body water, while obesity refers specifically to having an abnormally high proportion of body fat. Precisely measuring a person's body fat, however, is not easy. The most accurate method is to weigh person underwater, requiring expensive equipment in labs that are expensive and not convenient. Other methods for estimating body fat, such as skin fold thickness and bioelectric impedance analysis require a high degree of experience and can yield inaccurate results.

The most universally accepted indicator, accepted by health organizations around the world, is the body mass index [BMI] method. The BMI does not directly measure percent of body fat, but it provides a more accurate measure of overweight and obesity than relying on weight alone. The location of the body fat is also of concern and is measured separately. Generally women collect fat in their hips and buttocks, giving their figures a "pear" shape. Men, on the other hand usually build up fat around their bellies, giving them more of an "apple" shape. This measurement of fat location is called the waist –to-hip ratio. It is determined by measuring the waist at its narrowest point, then measuring the hips at the widest point, and dividing the waist measurement by the hip measurement.

Women with waist-to-hip rations of more than 0.8 or men with waist to hip rations of more than 1 are at increased health risk because of their fat distribution. A rule of thumb is that if a woman's waist measures more than 35 inches or a man's waist measures more than 40 inches they may be a particular risk for developing health problems. Studies indicate that increased abdominal or upper body fat is related to the risk of developing heart disease, diabetes, high blood pressure, gallbladder disease stroke and certain cancers. The location of body fat is also associated with overall mortality [likelihood of death]; whereas body fat concentrated in the lower body around the hips may be less harmful as a risk factor.

Body mass index

The National Institutes of Health [NIH] and the World Health Organization [WHO] basically agree and identify overweight as a BMI of 25-29 and obesity as a BMI of 30 or greater. Current evidence indicates that health risks increase more steeply in individuals with a BMI of 25 or more and trend to increase as the BMI increases. You can calculate your BMI by multiplying your weight in pounds times 700 and dividing that product by your height in inches squared. If you are not handy with math, tables of BMI are available from the NIH, and many health care providers. Some limitations for these methods may be that a senior who has lost muscle mass may be in the healthy weight category when they actually have reduced nutritional reserves. In other words BMI is a good general guideline but some individuals may have special considerations and require more sophisticated methods of body fat measurements.

Degree of **Disease Risks [1]**

Classification	BMI	Men- waist 40"or less Women – 35 in or less	Men-more than 40" Women-more than 35"
Underweight	Less than 18.5		
Normal	18.5 – 24.9		
Overweight	25 – 29.9	Increased	High
Obesity	30 -34.9	High	Very High
Obesity - II	35 – 39.9	Very High	Very High
Obesity -III	40 and more	Extremely High	Extremely High

[1]: Disease risk for type 2 diabetes, hypertension and CVD [cardiovascular disease]
Source: National Heart, Lung, and Blood Institute – NIH

Blood pressure (BP) is the force of blood against the walls of arteries. BP is Recorded as two numbers—the top number, the systolic pressure is measured as the heart beats and that number is recorded over the diastolic pressure (the relaxation of pressure as the heart relaxes between beats). For example, a blood pressure measurement of 120/80 mm Hg (millimeters of mercury) is expressed verbally as "120 over 80." Normal blood pressure is less than 130 mm Hg systolic and less than 85 mm Hg diastolic. However, optimal blood pressure is less than 120 mm Hg systolic and less than 80 mm Hg diastolic. Approximately 23 million U.S. adults with BPs in the high-normal range (systolic pressure of 130-139 mmHg and/or a diastolic pressure of 85-89 mmHg) are 1.5 to 2.5 times more likely to have a cardiovascular problem or die within 10 years, compared to those with optimal blood pressure, according to the Framingham Heart Study

5. How does America rate in world health?

American's have surprisingly high rates of premature death and disability when compared to many countries around the world. Previously, life expectancy estimates were based on the overall length of life compared to death rates in each country. However, that method included years that many people spend as disabled. Now The World Health Organization [WHO] calculates healthy life expectancy based on an indicator with the acronym of HALE, which stands for Health Adjusted Life Expectancy. "The HALE system is simple," explains Alan Lopez, M.D., Coordinator of WHO's Epidemiology and Burden of Disease Team. "In the old system, we measured total life expectancy based on the average numbers of year's males and females could expect to live in each country." However, people don't live all those years in perfect health. "At some point in your life, you will have some level of disability," continued Dr. Lopez. "These years with disability are weighted according to their level of severity to estimate the total equivalent lost years of good health." In other words, HALE adds up the number of years citizens of various countries are expected to be in "full health." To calculate HALE, the years of ill-health are weighted according to severity and then that figure is subtracted from the overall life expectancy to arrive at the equivalent years of healthy life.

Based on this new way to calculate healthy life expectancy, the Japanese have the longest healthy life expectancy in the world of 74.5 healthy years and shockingly, the U.S. is rated 24th under this system, with an average healthy lifespan of only 70 years. "The position of the United States is one of the major surprises of the new rating system," says Christopher Murray, M.D., Ph.D., director of WHO's Global Program on Evidence for Health Policy. "Basically, you die earlier and spend more time disabled if you're an American rather than a member of most advanced countries." Several factors combine to place various nations in the ranks of the worlds healthiest. One of the most important is the low rate of heart disease associated with the traditional low saturated fat diets eaten in those countries.

For example, Japan has only 29% of the U.S. rate for coronary heart disease (CHD), France had 38%, in 1997, and Italy in 1995 had 58%. Another factor is tobacco use. Countries, in which tobacco use is high, including the U.S., tend to come in low in the longevity rankings. Epidemiological studies [about 1960] also indicate that the traditional diets in Mediterranean countries such as Spain, Italy, and Greece are associated with healthy and long lived peoples. Medical evidence accumulated over the past three decades has documented that the low saturated fat, antioxidant phytochemical-rich diets of the Mediterranean countries and Australia, Japan, and China, have shown that the dietary patterns that prevail in these areas are "more important for longevity

Americans are ultra-conscious of their cholesterol readings. Many Americans know that the American Heart Association recommends keeping total cholesterol below 200, but not as many understand that there are two types of cholesterol, the "bad-guy" low density lipoproteins (LDL) that clog arteries causing atherosclerosis and the "good guy" high density lipoproteins (HDL) that actually are associated with a decreased probability of developing atherosclerosis. A recent study in the *British Journal of Nutrition* pointed out that the Mediterranean diet; especially the Greek version is dominated by the consumption of olive oil and by consumption of vegetables and fruits. Antioxidants represent a common element in these foods and antioxidant action provides a plausible explanation for the apparent benefits. Indeed, epidemiological data and the increasing understanding of their antioxidant mechanisms of action suggests that antioxidants play a major role in affecting in a beneficial way the health of the Mediterranean populations.

Study after study has suggested that red wine, a popular drink in the Mediterranean countries, such as France, Spain, and Italy, has cardio protective effects. Evidence, from a variety of sources has become overwhelming that a moderate intake of two glasses of wine, or other equal alcoholic drinks regularly helps prevent heart attacks. One recent study in the American Heart Association journal *Circulation* indicates that wine not only helps prevent heart disease, it also helps people who've already had one heart attack stop a second one. In that study, middle-aged men who had one heart attack and who drank two glasses of wine regularly were 50% less likely than nondrinkers to have a second heart attack, according to Dr. Michel de Lorgeril, of the Joseph Fourier University of Grenoble, France. More recent studies, appearing in the New England Journal of Medicine [2003], indicate that the type of alcohol beverage, whether wine, beer, or liquor was not significant in its reduction of the risk of myocardial infarction. While the most credible medical advice recognizes the health benefits from moderate drinking, it does not recommend that nondrinkers start drinking. The reasoning behind this is probably that nondrinkers may fail prey to the health risks of overdrinking, driving under the influences, etc.

Olive oil is important not only because of its own beneficial properties, but also because its use encourages the consumption of large quantities of vegetables and legumes in cooked meals and in salads. Since fat intake is required by the body, the use of olive oil with its monounsaturated properties fills this need without increasing one's chances for heart disease. In some of the Asia countries that have significant soy products in their diet, the level of certain kinds of cancer, such as breast and prostate, is less than one-third that in the U.S

6. Why this book is unique and credible

This book takes a unique three pronged approach to healthy weight loss

1. It recognizes that the underlying cause of the overweight and obesity is our obesity genes, encouraged by engineered foods. In response, it uses epigenetic modalities to modify or turn off our obesity genes.
2. It adopts the most proven eating program for healthy weight and longevity from the worlds healthiest and longest lived peoples [
3. It provides a diet that satisfies our obesity genes with healthy fats, sweets and quantity,

7. The Obesity Genes Diet [OGD]

Popular weight loss diets come and go, and from one aspect this is good, because many trendy diets are unhealthy. What is in vogue now will pass away and be resurrected at some later date, and all for a basic reason. Most of the trendy popular diets are not based on the science of clinic trails, but rather are only uninformed opinion. After all the hype and promotion on what's the best, the reality is that it is not the diet that fails but the lack of means to control our obesity genes.

In addition to the weight loss aspects, are the healthy longevity aspects. This aspect seems to get lost in the high focus on weight loss, mostly for the simple reason that healthy longevity doesn't sell. The large amount of studies performed by medical authorities, indicating that: low fat, fruits, vegetables, whole grains, and beans provide significant disease protection, gets ignored by the craze for fact weight loss, without giving up the popular Western diet. The bottom line is that dieting, without behavior changes, is always doomed to failure, because it connotes doing something unpleasant and unsatisfying, as well as fighting our instincts.

The Obesity Genes eating Plan

Researchers have long noted that the rates of heart disease, cancer, stroke, obesity, hypertension and diet differ widely in different geographic areas of the world. So what could be more obvious then to emulate the diets and lifestyles of the most successful? While it is agreed that observational studies don't necessarily prove cause and effect, the overwhelming number of studies and their concurrence make them the most logical plan as compared to popular diets that have no long term evidence. The OGD program is modeled on what the worlds longest lived and healthiest peoples eat and how they live. It is a plan that is rich in fruits, vegetables, and low-fat dairy products. It also reduces intake of saturated fat and sodium. And it is hardly a secret. The National High Blood Pressure Education Program in October updated its recommendations to just those types of foods. And, like our book, the NHBPEP recommends reducing excess body weight and increasing levels of physical activity. However, while they and virtually all the worlds' health organizations agree in theory, they fall short of fully recommending such diets, because they believe it would be unrealistic to think that most overweight and obese people could make such a significant change. And, limited to their self-discipline, that is evidently true. And therein lies the reason most diets fail long term. Most find that to fight their obesity genes' head on, is beyond their capabilities. Our book offers a comprehensive program of eating and genetic changes that can help you achieve those goals, by changing your beliefs and perceptions

The OGD eating program is modeled after the traditional diets of the world healthiest and longest lived peoples, before they trended to the Western type of diets. It also blends the healthiest foods from those diets, selecting those as compatible to Western tastes as possible. In addition, it takes into consideration new evidence from modern scientific studies, such as; certain foods in combination with certain medications; and recent environmental impacts of the quality of food, such as mercury levels in fish.

Features of the OGD

a. A natural plant-based diet is fundamental to all the HALL peoples, and is in opposition to the obesity gene driven food preferences of the high unhealthy fat and refined sugar nature of the Western diet. However, what tastes good is a learned habit and food preferences can be changed. EMP mental conditioning will help you change your subconscious food preference. This transition is made easier, since the Obesity Gene eating plan provides healthy fat, natural sweetness and unrestricted natural food calories. Hunger is not a problem with this eating plan since there are a variety of foods that have no limit. This is possible due the high nutrient density of vegetables and fruits, plus the morning and afternoon snacks.

b. For maximum convenience, there are flexible international menus for those have the time and desire for preparation; simple meals and snacks that anyone can put together from common staples available at any supermarket; and recommendations for restaurants and fast food outlets. Calorie counting is not required. A simple understanding of the types of foods that are healthy and those that are not, is sufficient.

c. We have many subconscious reasons for eating, such as stress, opportunity, emotional, and social that feed the motivation of our 'obesity genes'. The OGD eating program brings awareness to the opportunity for unnecessary eating.

d. The OGD is derived from the world's healthiest and longest-lived HALL peoples of the traditional Mediterranean countries, the elder Okinawa's, the traditional Japanese, and the rural Chinese. All of these have had the most extensive scientific nutritional clinical trials ever undertaken, on relating diet and disease, as well as longevity.

The most healthy features of each are blended together to give the 'best of the best'. Foods are prioritized relative to their associated disease protection, and recommended in the priority of; highest nutrient density, lowest GI, most fiber and the latest proven trials in scientific nutrition

8. Healthy Longevity of HALL peoples

The eating plan and lifestyles of the Healthy and Longed Lived [HALL] people have been verified by the largest and most comprehensive studies ever conducted. [See sources]

The following table indicates the significant difference in Heart Disease versus diet.

DEATH RATES PER 100,000 PEOPLE

LOCATION	DIET	LE *	CHD*
Okinawa	Asian	81.2	18
Japan	Asian	79.9	22
Hong Kong	Asian	79.1	40
Italy	Mediterranean	78.3	55
Greece	Mediterranean	78.1	55
U.S.	American	76.8	100

- LE – Life expectancy - CHD – Coronary Heart Disease
- Source is WHO [1996] and Japan Ministry of Health [1996]
- Does not include period of disability

The OGD eating plan is basically a blend from the following countries, enhanced with modern scientific studies and food availability,

a. The Traditional Mediterranean countries
b. Traditional Rural China
c. Traditional Okinawa Elders
d. Traditional Japan

WHO [World Health Organization] sponsored the MONICA project, the largest community-based study on heart disease ever undertaken, which studied the rates of heart disease among 170,000 people over a 10-year period. It showed that the lowest heart attack rates in females occurred in certain communities in Spain, China, France and Italy, as compared, for example, to Glasgow Scotland which had female heart attack rates eight times higher than in Catalonia, Spain. Among men, the lowest heart attack rates over the Ten year period were in certain communities in China, Spain, Switzerland and France. Citizens of North Karelia, Finland, on the other hand, had heart attack rates Ten times higher than those in Beijing, China.

The diets from these different regions with the lowest incidence of heart disease all have one main common denominator – They are based on natural plant foods as their major component. Their fat content may vary, but even then, the higher fat diets used fats from natural plant foods. Fundamentally, they all have a major part of the diet as complex carbohydrates, [natural plant foods] with a minimum amount of foods from animal products. One can argue the cause and effect nature, and what could have been and why this was, however it is a matter of history that a natural plant type of diet was associated with peoples that were healthier and longer lived then peoples whose diets were high in fatty animal foods and low in natural plant foods... The high-income, long-lived Japanese consume only about six percent of their calories from meat and seven percent from fish. In China, meat represents about eight percent of the diet. True, some of the Mediterranean peoples eat diets containing as high as 40% fat, but it is the healthy monounsaturated fat that comes from olive oil.

The OGD program emphasizes fruits, vegetables (often cooked in or flavored with olive oil) and whole grains as well as low-fat dairy foods, including butter substitutes (sterol food spreads) that taste like butter but are proven to reduce cholesterol, and nominal amounts of poultry, fish and lean meat. And yet we keep the most of the tastes desired by Americans with foods containing good fat, and natural sweetness. All these food products are combined into an array of delicious and tasty internationally oriented meals.

Instead of being new, trendy and unproven, the OGD eating plan is old, and proven healthier than the typical Western diet. It is not a departure into a new direction, but rather a return to healthier times. It is also compatible with the current recommendations of all the major medical and health care organizations, such as:

1. The American Institute for Cancer Research

The OGD formula has been shown in extensive studies by the American Institute for Cancer Research [AICR] as one of the main methods to reduce the risks of certain types of cancer. According to the AICR and its affiliate, the World Cancer Research Fund of the United Kingdom, more than 4,500 studies show a link between predominantly plant-based diets [vegetables, fruits and whole grains] and reduced cancer risk as well as reduced risks for many of the other diseases.

2. The World Health Organization
3. The American Medical Association
4. The National Institutes of Health
5. Major teaching institutions – Harvard, Mayo Clinic, Tufts, etc.

9. The OGD Bottom Line

We have presented an outline of the overwhelming body of evidence that the OGD eating plan has been proven by the HALL people, the longest and largest clinical studies, and he major World and American health organizations. These conclusions will be supported in more detail in later chapters. Assuming the argument will be reasonably proven, we can now logically put to rest all the arguments, concepts, opinions and theories promoted by the myriad of books, articles, the media, and other interests of what, and how much to eat for the best proven health and longevity. That is the easy part, since the basis of the OGD is a matter of history. What remains to find a method to reengineer ourselves to change our food preferences so that we want to eat what's better for us? To date, that has been the link. But now the new science of epigenetics solves that problem.

The goal of the OGD plan is a healthy weight loss of about 1/2 to 1 pound a week. A push for a rapid weight loss can disrupt the mental conditioning phase can undermine habit formation. Not only is a crash diet unhealthy but it is also unsustainable and will interrupt the development of a lifelong permanent change of eating patterns. We know from our studies of the world's healthiest people that a BMI of 18 to 24 is the natural, normal condition of those long-lived peoples. Remember, overweight is defined as a BMI of 25.0 to 29.9 and obesity is 30 or above. By shedding those unsightly extra pounds, you are protecting yourself from an assortment of diseases of aging and promoting healthy longevity.

The EMP program will be teaching you simple methods of mental conditioning using the tools of mindfulness, meditation, self-hypnotherapy and imagery to develop signals for healthier weight and longevity. Once you have conditioned your conscious mind to change your perceptions, epigenetic mechanisms will modify your obesity genes and you will enjoy your food preferences while maintaining a healthy weight. The same type of epigenetic programs that work for healthy weight can also be used with stress and pain management. The OGD will show you how to free your natural healing powers to bring about new eating and exercise patterns. You will learn to rewrite destructive eating and lifestyle scripts with your own conscious mind. The motivation of your obesity genes that have sabotaged your prior efforts at weight-control will lose their priority.

10. The Promises of This Book

In addition to healthy weight loss, this book will help you_live longer without disability because permanent weight-control and disease risk reduction link between overweight, obesity, diet and lifestyles to life threatening and disabling diseases. According to the World Health Organization (WHO), the fundamental causes for the obesity epidemic are changing behaviors, lifestyles, and eating habit over the past 20 years. In other words, we are becoming less physically active, living hectic, stress-filled lives, and are eating too much animal based foods and processed foods high in saturated and trans-fat fat, as well as refined sugar.

How fast can you lose weight?

Probably faster than advisable for health and long term change. According to the National Institutes of Health (NIH) guidelines, the initial goal of weight loss therapy is to reduce body weight by approximately 10 percent. A reasonable time line for a 10 percent reduction in body weight is six months of following the OGD. Once this goal is achieved, further weight loss can be attempted if more excess pounds have to be shed. (For overweight or obese patients with BMIs in the 27 to 35 range, a decrease of just 300 to 500 calories per day will result in the shedding of one-half to one pound of excess fat a week. Over a period of six months, that amounts to 12 to 24 pounds.

11. What Do You Have to Do?

1. The first step is to read and understand the concepts and evidence of the OGD eating plan. This will enable you to believe that it is founded on a sound basis and should work for you.
2. The next step is to get the attention of your conscious mind by becoming aware of your environment with the practice of mindfulness. Until you learn how to live in the present, your will be unable to achieve control of your conscious mind in order to make epigenetic changes.
3. Practice the epigenetic interventions of OGD self-hypnotherapy and imagery by following the scripts. With practice, you will be able to develop new eating habits to change your food preferences and eating habits. As a bonus, stress management will be facilitated by these techniques for mental conditioning.
4. You will also have to increase your physical activity levels, not only to burn more calories, but for general health and postponement of disabilities.

CHAPTER TWO

The genesis of our obesity epidemic

1. Introduction
2. Our 'obesity genes' under control
3. Our fat programming
4. Our sweetness programming
5. Our instinct for inactivity
6. The nature of our obesity genes
7. Genes out of sync
8. Our changing eating patterns
9. Our biological systems for bodyweight outmatched
10. Examples of encouraging our obesity genes
11. Epic changes in our environment in the latter part of the 20th century

    a. Family environment
    b. Inactivity
    c. Food Processing
    d. Levels of Development
    e. Psychological
    f. Food Consumer

1. Introduction

At our core, we are all products of our ancestors, changes in evolutionary forces and our life experiences. The degree that we are successful in survival and wellbeing is proportional to the degree that we are able to adapt to our environment. In a similar vein, our eating patterns have evolved to insure the survival of the species and the ability to pass on healthy genes to the next generation. Nature's design is efficient and unemotional. When the species is unable to adapt to a catastrophic environmental change, in time, the species is terminated. And this has been the case with the great majority of species that have been initiated and discontinued since life began. In the case of man, his unique capabilities have not only allowed faster adaptation, but also the ability to change his environment, which gives him the power to change the rules of the game of survival. But in the case of obesity, man's manipulation of the environment has had negative rather than positive effects. It is because we have changed our environment so drastically, in the latter half of the 20th century that our biological systems for body weight control are overwhelmed by our genetics. For want of a better term, for this natural genetic design for eating, I use the term 'obesity genes' to be self-descriptive and not too far away from the biology involved. As we shall see, it is the predisposition of our 'obesity genes' unrestrained and encouraged by our present drastically changed eating environment, that is the root cause of our skyrocketing obesity trend. In the following discussion, we shall see how this out of sync condition of early ancestor genes and present day environment came about to precipitate the present pandemic of overweight and obesity.

2. Our 'obesity genes' under control

Back in the days of our early ancestors, food was hard to come by. There were frequent times of shortages, due to weather, migrations, and environmental changes resulting in famines. Since the natural design our of our genetic programs is to insure survival as a first priority, genetic instructions, were to stock up on as many calories and fat reserves as possible to carry them through the hard times of food shortages. A similar situation is seen in animals putting on extra fat to get through the winter. Because plant foods, such as starchy roots, tubers, vegetables and fruit were the most available, they were the basic diet; however, fats and sweets were more prized because of their higher calorie density. However our early ancestors initially were only able to salvage injured or dead animals, until they were able to devise hunting and trapping methods. Because plant foods are low in calories, they had to keep eating throughout the day to stay alive, and the search for food was both exhausting and dangerous, requiring basically all of their time and energy. The combination of limited calories and high levels of physical activity maintained a healthy body weight. It doesn't require a stretch of the imagination to assume that there were few obese early ancestors.

3. Our fat programming

However, plant foods didn't provide the total solution, because biologically, the energy from plant foods is not storable for future needs, but is restricted to short term energy needs. The harsh demands of their environment required calorie reserves for protection during periods of food shortages. And the only food that that can be stored in our tissues is fat. To fill this need, our ancestors gorged themselves on any fat they came across. Some fats were available in certain plants, such as the seeds and nuts they could find in the fall, however, animal fats were the most desired source, and due to a lack of effective hunting weapons, they scoured the land for any dead or injured animal, attempting particularly before winter, to load up on fat. Filling up on the high calories in fat, became critical to survival, and since natural selection has to do with survival of the fittest, and you might say that in those days it meant survival of the fattest. Another feature of our fat programming is the ability of our body to reduce satiety when we eat fatty foods, which facilitates overeating and consequently storing more fat. This is compared to plant foods, which tend to be more filling on an equal calorie basis because of their higher volume and fiber

The genetic drive for fat was particularly critical for those with a less dependable

food supply, which is limited for migratory peoples. Recent studies tracking the DNA trails have shown that one of mans' migratory routes was from his cradle in Africa, through Asia, Siberia and across the Bering Straits to the Americas, facilitating 'obesity genes 'with plentiful food resources. A WHO press release [WHO/46.] June 97] showed that the prevalence of obesity in adults is 20 to 25% in the Americas, with a higher prevalence for obesity among American Indians, and Hispanic Americans. Another migratory route led to the Pacific Islands, which today has one of the highest obesity rates. Among the Melanesians, Micronesians and Polynesians, the obesity rates are about for 70% for women and 65% for men.

4. Our Sweetness programming

In addition to our fat programming, our 'obesity genes' also have a sweetness preference. It is logically assumed that our instinct for sweetness originally evolved to prefer fruits and other carbohydrates that were the sweetest and consequently the most mature and calorie laden. Carbohydrates come in two forms, complex carbohydrates and simple sugars. Complex carbohydrates are long chained sugar molecules, wrapped in fiber and water. When you eat complex carbohydrates, such as whole grains, vegetable or fruit the digestive process is extensive in order to separate the sugars from the fibers. This lengthy process requires an extended digestive tract in order to be able to perform the efficiently, which would suggest that our lengthy digestive tract confirms our design as a basic plant eater. Many other physical features, such as our type of teeth, further confirm that we are basically designed to eat plants. When the sugar is separated it is absorbed by the small intestine, to enter our bloodstream where it can be used as fuel or stored in the liver or muscle as glycogen... Since this process is lengthy and essential a low flow process it provides a longer lasting energy. The nature of complex carbohydrates in natural plant foods is that they are low in calories and slowly absorbed over many hours, making it available when quick energy is needed. Another feature of carbohydrates, particularly in fruits, is that when they are undeveloped that are less sweet then when they are mature and ripe, and present the best nutrition. It is thought that this 'sweet tooth' in our ancestors evolved as the virtually universal craving of children for candy. At any rate, we don't need a lot of research to convince us of the universal desire for sweetness. Unfortunately most of this desire is filled today by products loaded with unnatural and unhealthy refined carbohydrates.

5. Our instinct for inactivity

Loading up on calories, was made simpler by our programming to burn less calories. Consequently, it is believed that our early ancestors' experienced a natural decrease of their metabolic rate when they were unable to eat sufficient food. This conserved energy, since metabolic rate determines how fast calories are burned as energy. Since physical activity exercise increased the requirement for energy they would also reduce their activity as much as possible consistent with that required to survive and multiply. This instinct is easily observable in our lifestyles of today and many studies show the increasing trend of reduced physical activity by increasing automation and labor saving devices.

6. The nature of our obesity genes

In researching the genes most responsible for bodyweight regulation, experiments With animals have shown that if the appetite gene is incapacitated, animals continue to eat normally, however, if the satiety gene is incapacitated, an animal will eat insatiably. Taking another tack, scientists have long been searching for the appropriate genes to increase our metabolism, until it was recently determined that the obese have a higher metabolism then average, which removed the interest in this approach. One type of genetic research that has been substantially proven on a variety of animals, and even primates is that significant calorie restriction increases life span, on the order of a 30% calorie reduction results in a 30% increase in life span. While this may be suitable for animals, few humans will put up with a reduction of calories of that order.

Our genetic programming features present a barrier to conventional diet attempts for restrictive dieting. When you start reducing calories, our body senses this is famine and responds by slowing our metabolic rate to compensate, which offsets the effect of calorie restriction on weight loss. If you continue to reduce your calorie consumption or miss meals, you will experience hunger pains and possibly even more symptoms such as fatigue, weakness, shaky limbs, anxiety and a strong craving for fatty types of foods. A situation no many of us will endure for long. The genome, [our total genetic code] is often described as our genetic programming, but it is not like the typical computer program. Rather than a rigid computer program, not all genetic designs are behavioral commands. But rather predisposition's that are like a voice whispering in your ear to do it, but yet we can make another choice. In order for genes to motivate a response, they have to be activated, which is not always the case. A well know example is in the case of identical twins that although they have identical genomes, have differences personalities due the epigenetic link with since different perceptions.

The natural selection concept of evolution theory, tells us that not all genes are equal.

Witness the families we all know where most of them are overweight and yet one is lean, or in the opposite case of identical twins, raised in different environments, but yet both tend to the same body weight. One of the first breakthroughs occurred in 1995 when a hormone produced by fat cells caused fat to melt away in mice. This hormone was termed leptin and recently other compounds that have the power to regulate appetite have been discovered. The hypothalamus activated by the hormone leptin for related chemicals directs the energy use of the cells and tissues. And the body responds by idly fidgeting in order to raise metabolic rates and increase blood flow to the outer layers of the skin in a process called thermogenesis. In order to dissipate excessive calories. Leptin influences appetite and thermogenesis in maintaining our energy balance. As we put on more fat, leptin increases to signal the hypothalamus to accelerate energy output and slow caloric intake. Unfortunately, people who have the tendency to gain weight are showing a remarkable resistance to the power of leptin. The fatter they get the more leptin they make, the more impervious the hypothalamus becomes. In time the hypothalamus reads the elevated level of leptin as normal and misreads the drop in leptin as a starvation signal. This biomechanism is an explanation for why so many of those who lose weight end up putting it back on. Our 'obesity genes' backed by millions of years of evolution, fight us at every turn.

A joint Swiss-German-American Study, reported in the New England Journal of Medicine in March of 2003 makes one of the strongest cases yet that genetic changes can cause an eating disorder. For decades, researchers have been trying to understand the reasons for the present epidemic of obesity. About 30 % of American Adults are obese up from 14 percent 25 years ago and the surge is widely blamed on abundant high-calorie foods and sedentary lifestyles. However some researchers have also begun to link several genes to obesity, implicating heredity as an important underlying factor. Increasingly eating problems are thought to stem from a subtle interaction of lifestyle land multiple genes. Probably the most common eating disorder, binge-eating strikes up to 4 million Americans. In this study, the researchers focused on the melanocortin 4 receptor genes, which make a protein by that name that helps stimulate appetite in the brain's hunger-regulating hypothalamus. If a mutated gene makes too little protein, the body feels too much hunger. According to this study, the binge eating syndrome tied to this gene is perhaps; the most stubbornly resistant to dieting and exercise.

The non-technical term 'obesity genes' is comprised of at least the following actions as our hunger hormones work in sequence to regulate eating. Some of the initial hormones discovered include: **PYY3-36** - released by cells in the digestive tract in response to food. This hormone tells the brain the body is full. **GHRELIN** - When the stomach is empty. Its cells release ghrelin, a hormone that brings on hunger pangs. **INSULIN** - The master regulator of the amount of glucose in the blood, insulin is secreted by the pancreas and determines how much glucose in burned off-and how much is stored as fat. **CHOLECYSTOKININ**- Once the food reaches the small intestine; this hormone triggers the release of digestive enzymes and acts as a signal to stop eating. **LEPTIN** -a hormone secreted by fat cells in the body, it keeps fat levels constant. A lot of leptin in the blood leads to a drop in appetite and more rapid calorie burning. Genes by themselves don't make us fat, but unrestrained by an encouraging environment they take their toll. Our sedentary lifestyles and a cornucopia of animal based and refined carbohydrates have made Americans the equivalent of corn-fed cattle confined in pens.

7. Genes out of sync

Our 'obesity genes' are not the only ones out of sync with the present environment. Whenever our biological design is suited for one or a set of environmental conditions and the environment or conditions substantially change at a rate faster than the evolutionary process, our genes are out of 'sync'. Another of the classic examples of genes out of sync is our 'fight or flight' response, during which hormones like adrenaline and cortisol are released, causing our metabolism, heart rate, blood pressure, breathing rate and muscle tensions all to increase. In the environment of our early ancestors this was a very handy response, to prevent being eaten by a saber tooth tiger, or attacked by a relative who's hungry for our food, and other such threats to survival. However, times have changed and evolution is long behind catching up, making this 'fight or flight' response usually inappropriate today.

In the case of our 'obesity genes', we no longer are endangered by food shortages, [at least in affluent countries], in fact quite the opposite, we are overwhelmed by food abundance, stuffed with high density calories. Our obesity genes, which were lifesavers at one time in history, now are just the opposite, contributing to making us fatter and fatter and sicker and more disabled. Likewise for the 'flight or fight' response. When the response occurs repeatedly, such as in chronic stress, it can have detrimental effects on the body. Such as contributing to heart disease with high levels of cortisol suppressing the immune system. Most medical authorities agree that stress plays a part in virtually all physical and mental disease and dysfunction. On an acute level, its effects can be seen every day, not only in world conflicts, but as road rage, brawls, physical and mental abuse and on and on.

8. Our changing eating patterns

The evolution of our eating patterns has been formed by climate, geography culture, industrialization, technology, affluence and other circumstances. The Three basic classifications of food systems are the **Gatherer-Hunter,** which goes back to prehistoric times, the **Peasant - Agricultural**, which began about 10,000 years ago and the **Urban-Industrial** system, which is very recent.

Gatherer-Hunter

Anthropological findings and recent studies of isolated groups, suggest they subsisted by gathering fruits, such a berries and plants, such a leaves and tuber and legumes together with meat obtained by scavenging and hunting. It is generally thought that the gathering of plant foods was a greater part of their diet then the meat from hunted animals, with fish and seafood more important in the coastal areas. A taste for sweetness evolved probably because of its indication that fruits are ripe and that plant foods are safe to eat, and a taste for fat the most energy dense food, became a matter of survival in times of food shortage, such as in winter and during migration.

Peasant-Agricultural

People living in the Middle East region over 10,000 years ago, discovered that cereals could be grown and processed to cook as bread or dried. This development permitted feeding larger groups of people, forming growing communities. The types of different grains were adapted in regions generally where the climate was most conducive to its cultivation. While domesticated animals have been bred for food for thousands of years, usually only the wealthy ate any significant amounts

Urban-Industrial

The industrial revolution interrupted the evolution of natural diets as food supplies in North American and Europe in the nineteenth century produced food on mass scale, of which much use to be common only in the diets of wealthy people. With the invention of the steel roller mills, in the 1870s, white bread, and other refined cereal products, containing lower levels of fiber, essential oils, vitamins and minerals then whole grain, was commonly available. Sugar refined from cane was a valuable cash crop, and led to the development of the biscuit, cake, chocolate, confectionery, jam and soft drink industries. Railways made it possible for vast tracts of American to be used for rearing cattle and the growth of the meat industry, and fatty meat became everyday food for most. With the discovery in the nineteenth century that animal protein promotes growth, the US established a network of agricultural universities to foster meat and dairy science as the foundation of nutrition. As one result, production of fatty meat was increased as livestock were fed with cereals previous used as human food rather then left to grazing on marginal lands. Consumption of fat rose in the industrial world in the twentieth century partly as a result of meat as an everyday staple and the increase in full fat milk, cheese and butter. The hydrogenation process was developed in the early twentieth century to provide improved food processing, and also resulted in an entirely new fat source, called trans-fats.

Due to these changes, the diets eaten in economically developed countries and urban areas became relatively low in cereals, tubers and other starchy foods, and relative high in sugar, fat, animal protein, salt, meat, dairy products and alcohol. As countries became industrialized, starchy staples decreased from 50% or more of total energy intake to 25% or less, and fat increased from less the 20% to 40% of total energy intake. Consequently, diets generally become more energy dense and people became more sedentary as industrialization required less physical labor, and as a result, the seeds for the current world pandemic of overweight and obesity where sown. Consumption of vegetables and fruits became more a function of climate and availability than of culture, such as in the Mediterranean region. Refrigerated distribution systems allowed consumption in relatively rich industrial regions.

Current eating patterns

According to a World Cancer Research Fund/American Institute for Cancer Research. Extensive study on 'Food, Nutrition and the prevention of cancer' and a Food and Agriculture Organization of the United Nations study on 'Protein quality evaluation', eating patterns are significantly evolving as countries develop. Food groups are changing in patterns such as Africa and Asia [excluding Japan] where half or more of total energy is supplied by cereals, whereas in Europe and North American less than one quarter of total energy is supplied by cereals. Consumption of added fats, alcohol, meat, dairy products and sweeteners is generally inverse to consumption of starchy staples. In the economically developed world more than 15% of total energy comes from meat, whereas in the economically developing world it is less than 10% and in some cases it is much less. On a global basis from 1960 to 1990 the general tendency is for consumption of cereal foods to decrease and added fats, alcohol, meat and dairy produce to increase with consumption of total fats is increasing in all regions of the world, while vegetables and fruits showing little change.

Cereals are the staple food of most Asian countries as a function of income. The highest levels being in low-income countries, for instance in China cereals amount to 69%. Asian diets, in middle to low income countries, are low in fats, containing few animal foods, and vegetables and fruits are generally found only in high-income areas. . The high income Japanese consumes only about 6% in meat and 7% in fish. In China meat represents about 8%. The trend data for Asia in 1960-1990 reflects the food groups typically associated with rapid industrialization and urbanization. Most countries show a decrease in cereal consumption except for low-income countries. The most affluent show an increase in vegetables and fruits, and substantial increases in the intake of meat and dairy products. However, their meat and dairy product consumption is still low in comparison to US diets.

Countries known as the Mediterranean countries [Greece, Italy, France, Portugal, Spain, and former Yugoslavia] for many years have had diets somewhere between the traditional rural and industrial patterns. In the early part of the 20th century their diets were low in meat and high in cereal, [mostly wheat] vegetables and fruits, tuber and pulses. Fish also was a significant part, particularity for those near coastal areas. The most unique feature of their diet was that they derived most of their fats from the high use of olive oil. Currently, cereals, [mostly wheat] provide about 25% of their total energy, with edible fats and oils contributing about 19%. Total dietary fats, milk and dairy products contribute about 35 to 40% and meat products an average 15%. Vegetables and fruits are consumed in appreciable quantities in all southern Europe on average of 6% with sweeteners about 9% and alcohol consumption is high and ranges from 8% in Portugal to about 3% in Greece. From 1960 to 1990 cereal consumption has declined by an average of 30%, and milk and dairy products, scarcely consumed in the past have substantially increased. Consequently, dietary fat has increased greatly, from 160% in Greece to a low of 20% in France. Countries with the highest percent changes are those that in the past had the lowest consumption of meat, such as

Italy, Spain and Portugal. This trend in the Mediterranean countries over the last 30 years from less cereals and more fat is most likely a significant factor in increasing their previous global low level of heart disease.

American diets are diverse and not predominated by a single food group. Cereals attribute 23%, and are most consumed as; biscuits crackers, breakfast cereals cakes and pastries, which also contribute hidden fats, oils and sweeteners to the diets. Edible fats and oils contribute 18%, sweeteners 16%, milk products 15%, and dairy products about 10%. Total dietary fats total about 37% with vegetables and fruits about 6%. For the period of 1960-90, intakes of cereals, meats and total fats have remanded stable whereas vegetables and fruit has increased about 10 to 20% and milk and dairy declined about 20-30%. The saturated fatty acid content of the diet fell about 15-20% and alcohol increased substantially about 30%. While total dietary fat has decreased in recent times, it has been more than replaced by more calories and hidden trans-fats in so called low-fat processed foods, fast foods, opportunistic eating and 'value sized' portions. Consequently, the trend toward more high-density calories and more sedentary couch time has fueled the American epidemic of overweight and obesity.

From prehistory to the 20th century, the balance between our 'obesity genes' and environment was generally in 'sync' and body-weight was reasonably healthy. Throughout this period, food was usually scarce and chiefly consisted of plant based foods and required considerable work to get it. Then in the early part of the 20th century, Americans started environmental changes that set off events that precipitated present times. At that time, Great Britain was working to solve a problem of the working classes getting shorter and leaner. Working in new field of nutrition, scientists thought they had discovered the necessary nutrients to solve the problem. Their studies suggested that milk or meat supplements made children grow taller and sturdier, and public pressure soon forced government programs to support the production of milk and meat. This movement started to spread among similar cultures, like the

US. Shortly thereafter, WW1 came along and preventing a shortage of food supply became a priority. The incentive to process food that could be stored for long periods and produced in large supply spawned the food processing industry that has grown to dominate our dietary patterns.

To prevent food rationing during World War II, agricultural policy emphasized the product of milk and meat as a matter of national survival. Since World War II, food production was the order of the day for developed countries all over the world and science responded with new efficient farming methods with pesticides, growth regulation, genetic selection and more efficient production of livestock and dairy herds. Food processing started to really take off after WWII when packaged food was viewed as a cheap and efficient way to feed the population. They were often 'enriched' and there was no real concern, that they contained high fat and sugar content, preservatives, and a variety of relatively untested chemicals to aid processing and storage. The fact that the products had good quantities of calories and a blend of nutrients believed to promote good health seem to be a reasonable approach to the nutritional knowledge of those days. The reality of an advancing technology and vastly automated society, with its less labor intensive demands, requiring less calories was not taken into consideration. And it has only later that we realized that highly processed and packaged food, in addition to questionable additives, and a deficiency of phytochemicals and fiber, sometime contains too many calories, sugar and fat. Meanwhile, the US emphasized meat and dairy products, and process foods, while peoples in certain other countries, particularly in Asia and the Mediterranean countries continued on their traditional basic natural plant food orientation with minimal animal products. The HALL peoples continued to enjoy the highest levels of health and lowest incidence of heart disease, stroke, forms of cancer and a number of other debilitation diseases in the world. Again reminding us, that as so often is the case, man's manipulation of our environment often has results not contemplated that greatly outweigh any conceived benefits.

While it had often been stated that obesity is a complex condition, one with serious social and psychological dimensions, the fact is that the obesity epidemic is not just rampant in industrialized societies, but also is those that those that are developing and even in societies that are still comparatively primitive. While the environment in the higher developed countries is prone to lessen the reins on the obesity genes the fact of a genetic underpinning gives rise to increasing bodyweight is all societies. It's only the degree that is varies. The mammoth environmental changes imitated early in the 20th century have allowed us the immediate pleasure brought about by eating palliative foods and reduced physical activity, but at a cost that far exceeds the benefits.

To sum up, while there are certainly stories and records of obese people throughout recorded history, percentages of overweight and obesity were nominal compared to the percentages today and most of these were of the more affluent, where rich foods were available without physical effort. At any rate there is no record of large numbers of fat peasants. Since clinical trials are not available, epidemiology, observation and reasoning are our best tools to the likely theory that the combination of natural plant type foods and physical activity that were the hallmark of yesteryear and nonexistent in the America of today, are the bonds that restrained our obesity genes. This line of reasoning is bolstered the following evidence.

a. According to the World Health Organization, the world's HALL peoples, [primarily Mediterranean and Asian countries] were all plant and fish eaters, physically active and lean. While this was the case with their traditional diets and lifestyles to about 1960, the trending towards the so called 'Western diets' and lifestyles has begun to significantly erode their earlier healthier status .

b. A number of examples of isolated cultures that were plant and fish eaters and healthy, active and lean that quickly became obese and disease ridden when abundant rich food, without work, became suddenly available.

c. The concurrence of the US obesity epidemic, the US policymakers focus on meat, dairy products and processed food, and other significant changes in our eating environment, such as our accelerating level of development. This and a rising level of affluence provided more opportunity to partake of the overabundance of rich, processed and fast foods. This was coupled with a rapid increase in leisure and technology, and a corresponding decrease in physical activity and manual labor provided ample opportunity to overeat and vegetate.

d. Ironically, at the same time, our increased level of development demanded a faster pace of life, 2 workers in a family, more stress and less disposable time for healthy eating, putting a priority on fast and effortless meals foods.

In other words, there were a contributing number of events and changes in our environment that resulted in consuming more unhealthy calories and less physical activity.

9. Our biological systems for bodyweight outmatched.

Until our environment took a sudden turn to the right, in recent decades, as discussed above, our homeostatic mechanism for our weight control historically maintained a relatively healthy body weight. First a simple discussion of how we are designed to work, when nature was in total control of our environment. Our biological control center of hunger is a network of organs throughout the body whose key structure is the hypothalamus and related structures. Hunger is regulated by two systems. One is a feeding system that initiates eating when food is needed and the second is a satiety system that stops eating when enough food has been consumed. The information the hypothalamus uses in regulating hunger are;

Stomach contractions - The most immediate cue in the regulation of hunger comes from the stomach. Contraction signal the feeding system, while a full stomach activates the satiety system.

Blood Sugar Levels - Eating is also regulated on a short-term basis by the amount of sugar [glucose] in the blood. The liver detects glucose levels that fallen below the level needed to provide energy to the body cells and sends messages to the feeding center in the hypothalamus that initiate hunger and eating. In addition, the upper small intestine reacts to sugar in the food that has been eaten and sends messages to the satiety center of the hypothalamus that lead to the end of hunger. In addition the hypothalamus contains specialized neurons that can detect the level of glucose in the bloodstream. This has been demonstrated in three major ways.

a. When insulin in injected into the bloodstream of a satiated person, it cause a drop in the level of glucose and the person feels hunger

b. When the hormone glucagon is injected into the bloodstream of a hungry person, it increases blood glucose and reduce hunger. Blood glucose levels are a key mechanism in the control of hunger. Since it takes a little time for food to be digested and enter the bloodstream in the form of glucose, dieters are often advised to eat more slowly to reach a level of blood glucose that makes them feel "full" before they reach their accustomed level of food intake

c. Blood fat levels - The long term maintenance of body weight is managed by a different mechanism. The hypothalamus is thought to monitor the level of the fat glycerol in the blood. When an individual gains weight, blood glycerol increases. The hypothalamus then restores long term body weight by signaling a decrease in hunger or an increase in activity level that would burn off calories or both. This homeostasis mechanism acts as a set point for the body, and it is difficult to raise or lower body weight above or below this set point for very long by sheer will power.

d. Psychological influences biological - while the above discussions on the biological set point for body weight is an underlying element of human biological design, it obviously is not absolute, since it can be overridden by new habits, motives and emotions produced by a number of psychological factors. For instance, learning and culture have a large influence on what, how much and when we eat. Emotions also play a role in eating. For example people who are anxious often may under or over eat more than usual and those who are depressed may lose their appetite all together. One of the most concerning psychological factors are stimuli that activate the genes which override our normal hunger regulation. For instance, seeing or smelling one of your favorite foods, even when you fill full can stimulate your hypothalamic to release insulin which stimulates hunger by causing your blood sugar to drop

10. Examples of encouraging our obesity genes.

As discussed we are genetically predisposed to eat more calories, fats and sweets then are healthy for our present environment. Mutations in our genes and our individual environment, basically determines our level of predisposition and where we fall on a continuum from a healthy bodyweight to obesity. This is not a unique theory, growing scientific thought now believes genetic programs predispose us to obesity and it's only the type and strength of our environmental restrictions that can prevent or allow that condition. As previously discussed, these genetic programs to overeat, were held in check by limited food availability, natural types of mostly plant foods, fish and limited meat, and considerable physical activity to bring the food to the table, and our biological weight maintenance systems. Up until the mid-20th century, these environmental limiters were sufficient to regulate a healthy body weight, but when high energy food becomes available just for the asking and without the need for physical activity, the results are dramatic. Such an example, of genetics forces unleashed by sudden removal environmental restraints, was dramatically played out in micro scale of a South Sea Island.

Until recently, Koskae, a small Micronesia island in the South Pacific enjoyed their traditional unsophisticated culture, using substantial manual labor to harvesting the local fruits and vegetables, supplemented by fishing. The people were healthy, relatively long lived and non-communicable diseases where rare. Then one day, the US showed up trading substantial dollars to buy access to their island for military purposes. Along with the new affluence, the natives were introduced to the high energy and unhealthy foods of Westernization. It wasn't long before they were importing plenty of canned fatty meats, dairy products, processed foods, soda, candy, potato chips and a wide variety of other junk food. And to top it off, they didn't have to do any work to get it, other than to open the cans and boxes. In a remarkably short time, their innocent culture was destroyed and obesity ran rampant, taking victims of over 75% of the population. Along with the obesity, unhealthy foods and lack of exercise came; heart disease, high blood press, diabetes, cancer and strokes. Today, the islanders typically die in their 50ies, accepting their fate, and not interested in a return to their traditional culture. While this is only one example, and admittedly the 'obesity genes' might well be stronger due to the migratory inheritance of their ancestors, there are many other examples of peoples becoming westernized by relocation, increasing levels of development, etc. Another example in macro scale can be seen by comparing the high world health ranking of the Mediterranean and Asian countries some 40 to 50 years ago to their present deteriorated ranking, as their traditional diet and life styles became more westernized.

An example of the same trend, but at a different rate, is illustrated by the so called 'French Paradox'' What is clear from the above study on a South Sea Island, Mediteranean and Asian countries and elsewhere is that not every culture has the same 'strength' of 'obesity genes'. For example, the French have demonstrated an unusual ability to keep a normal bodyweight, and low incidence of heart disease in spite of a reputation for extensively rich foods. This unusual situation is well known as the 'French paradox' and is frequently explained away as due to their red wine. However, there is no conclusive proof of this, and it seems like a case of rationalization, conceivably initiated by the French wine industry. It is more likely, that the 'Paradox' can be explained more reasonably by the comparatively few calories the French eat, as anyone who has traveled in France can attest. As to why their culture has inherited mutated weak 'obesity genes' is not known. It would seem likely that they descended from a culture that was not subjected to frequent food shortages and famine. While they are most likely to be genetically disposed, not to overeat, and among the leanest in the developed world, they still have traces of 'obesity genes' as almost 10% of French adults are now overweight.

Another example of our 'obesity genes' in action is found in two groups of Pima Indians, one living in Arizona and the other in Mexico's Sierra Madre Mountains. The Pimas' in Arizona have long been known for high rates of obesity and diabetes [almost 50%] The Mexico Pimas' where food is sparser and manual labor more common tend to be lean, and have a much lower rate of obesity and diabetes, but still higher than the general population.

11. Epic changes in our eating environment in the latter part of the 20th century

    a. Family Environment
    b. Inactivity
    c. Food Processing
    d. Levels of Development
    e. Psychological
    f. Food Consumerism

a. Family Environment

From an environmental viewpoint, obesity commonly has its start in childhood. It is then when the habits of eating patterns and physical activity are influenced by their parents, schools, TV, video games, processed and junk foods, authoritative figures, etc. We are born with only a few taste prejudices; an aversion to bitter, hot or sour and a preference for fat, sweet and salt. The rest of our food preferences are basically learned. Our children's' environment has changed so drastically in the past two decades, that their unrestricted 'obesity genes' are having a field day.

In just two decades, overweight and obesity in American children has more than doubled, and childhood obesity in the US has skyrocketed from about 5 percent in 1964 to triple that in 1999. This swelling trend is not unique to the western world, as it is the same story for the other developed and developing countries. For instance, in Britain, youth obesity rates soared by 70 percent in a single decade. With this trend comes the diseases it brings, for instance, children now amount to about 30% of all diagnosed cases of diabetes. Subconscious programs that predispose the children toward obesity are difficult to overcome, and frequently stay with the child into early childhood and into adolescence become reinforced in neural pathways. For example, an overweight child at 2 years has a reasonable chance at normal weight if their genetically driven subconscious unhealthy eating programs are restrained. However, by the time they reach 15, their unhealthy eating habits are frequently too deeply ingrained to resist and adult obesity is usually the result. Frequent studies and research identify too many hours before the TV as one of the most serious risks for overweight, not just because of the inactivity, but also because of the snacking of junk foods that usually accompanies the viewing. Studies show that that a typical child, around the age of 10, spends about 5 inactive hours [including PC or video games] a day in front of the TV, with its suggestive high proportion of high-fat food commercials. And frequently, high fat snacks are also in attendance and now account for about 20 % of their daily calories.

To make the matter worse, frequently TV commercials encourage eating of the sponsors products, which are not usually foods that suit their genetic programming for fats, sweets and overeating. High on the list for marketing to children are junk foods such as soft drinks, candy bars, sugary breakfast cereals and a wide range of fast foods. These types of foods are also frequently part of school menus, and are available in vending machines at schools and elsewhere. Since the opportunity to eat genetically favored foods is promoted on TV, in the movie lobbies, endorsed by our schools and allowed by their

families, what is a kid to think, other than it is OK. By the time the child reaches the age where they can think for themselves, it's usually too late to resist the powerful unhealthy subconscious programs that are deeply etched in their brains. The environment of the unhealthy nutrition at their schools, in combination with the reduced schedules for athletics and restricted physical activity present a powerful message to an impressionable child that junk food and inactivity are the way to live.

The child unknowing is led by the authority figures in their life, into a lifelong fight against the effects of reduced quality of life, and the diseases that are linked to overweight and obesity. According to The U.S. center for Disease Control and Prevention, children obesity has doubled since 1965. The consequence of this is that the child has a 40% chance of being overweight or obese and an 80% chance if both parents are overweight. The fact that 1965 is selected as a point of reference is not indicative that there was no stimulus for overweight before then. As discussed previously, the starting point for a more accelerated environment change was initiated in the first world war period with the move away from natural foods towards meat, dairy products, and the processing and marketing of 'simulated foods'.

b. Inactivity

From our early ancestors to recent times in the 20th century, humans have managed to maintain a relatively healthy body-weight by keeping sufficiently physically active to offset our calorie intake. But in recent times when our activity has drastically diminished, in general, our body weight has increase somewhat in proportion. Those who are somewhat less possessed by their obesity genes manage more to escape this law of nature, but that's not the case for the majority of us. Ever increasingly, technology with its labor saving widgets and processing speed drives the business activities that used to be performed by our physical effort. In the 1950's activity was an integral part of daily life while today, there are few manual jobs, a labor -saving device for every task and a preference to spend leisure time watching TV.

While technology produces higher productivity and more efficient and profitable business, it does so necessarily by using more brain and less body. Unfortunately, as we become less active, our appetite does not get reduced proportionally and our subconscious programs still drive for the calories, resulting in their storage as fat.

According to the National Institutes of Health [NIH] only 22 percent of U.S. adults get the recommended regular physical activity during non-work time, of 5 times a week for at least 30 minutes of any intensity. And maybe bout 15 percent get the recommended amount of vigorous activity of 3 times a week for at least 20 minutes. About 25 percent of adults claim they don't do physical activity at all during their non-work time. This level of physical activity palls in comparison to that performed by the world healthiest and longest lived peoples.

c. Food Processing –from natural to simulated

One of the more obvious environmental changes is that in the developed and developing areas of the world there is little concern for a lack of food, and ironically we are threatened by an overabundance which presents its own host of dangers. Intensifying this threat is that this overabundance has been developed technologically to produce a profit rather than the health of the user. In order to do this, the product must have a 'value added' When a plant food is processed it may be altered by a multitude of means, some examples are; pulverizing, milling, juicing, refining, dehydrating, and reconstituting. These processes remove the fiber and water and many nutrients resulting in a source of more concentrated, and less healthy calories. To put back the nutrients, they take out, they are enriched [a marketing term] by adding ingredients that supposed reconstitute their natural form, and then some. In addition, there are added a host of unnatural chemicals, including fat and sweetness for taste, preservatives for extended shelf life, ease of processing, and cost reduction. In addition, other chemicals are added to enhance marketing, increase profit margins and east of manufacture. The result of all this manipulation results in less nutrition then natural foods, and with a higher density of calories.

For example, consider the calorie density is found in the case of a white potato. A medium size potato has about 440 calories, and weighs about one half pound. If it is processed into French fries, it now has about 600 calories. Then if more oil is added to turn it into a half pound of potato chips, it now has about 1,300 calories. The results are more than triple the natural calories with a generous supply of artery plugging fat. Obviously this appeals to the American public, since one-third of the vegetables eaten in the US are either French fries or potato chips.

Our fuel ratio

Normally, we roughly burn an equal fuel mix of both fat and carbohydrates. However, when we eat a significant amount of processed carbohydrates, we absorb a higher level of sugars [carbohydrates] which must be burned, since they can't be stored, and accordingly more fat must be stored. For maximum nutrition and health body weight, the world's healthiest and longest lived peoples feast on natural complex carbohydrates whereas the majority of Americans fast on simple carbohydrates. The consumption of sugar and white flour in processed foods has trended steeply upwards in the past few decades, instep with obesity trend. When whole grains were refined for ease of processing and preservation, is the day when we started to move from natural body weight to the larger 'processed' body weight. Since then, feeding our obesity genes from the simple carbohydrates in refined grains, cakes, white bread, bakery, etc. rather than the natural whole grains in complex carbohydrates appears to be one part of the formula for a swelling body weight, and its linked diseases.

The problems of sugar overload

High levels of sugar, such as from processed carbohydrates, because our pancreas to produce corresponding levels of the hormone insulin, and in the process, increases our appetite. Because they don't have the fiber and water of plant foods, a large volume can be eaten before the stomach's receptors signals that you are getting full and shutting off your appetite... Insulin acts to permit your cells to utilize the sugar as fuel or store it as glycogen in your muscles and liver, if room is available. If it isn't, then the excess blood sugar is burnt as fuel. However, as mentioned above, our normal fuel mixture is about 50% sugar and 50% fat, and burning high levels of sugar, causes the fat that normally would be burned to be stored in our tissues. On the other hand, consuming natural plant foods, the sugar intake is reduced and we are then able to burn fat in order to meet our energy needs. The control of our insulin is obviously necessary to facilitate the optimum fuel mixture so that we burn fat instead of storing it. And the most efficient way to do that is to eat complex rather than simple carbohydrates, keeping the calories and insulin level low to burn fat, thus preventing its storage.

Low fat doesn't necessary mean less bodyweight

In recent times the American public finally started to take the bad PR on low fat seriously, generating an unfilled need for more low fat foods. The food processors, happy to comply, came out with a number of processed foods label 'low fat'. However, this was a false start because when they just took out the fat, the obesity genes weren't happy with the unfamiliar and unpalatable taste, and the American public indicated their displeasure by closing their pocketbooks. So the food processors did some brain storming on the quandary of how to remove fat and still taste like fat and came up with some marketing tricks. One was to increase the size of the meal by adding some fat free food, [such as fat free desert] so that they could label the total meal with a lower percentage of fat. This allowed more fat in the basic part of the meal and still got under the bar. The fat free portion usually contained a high level of sugar to satisfy the sweetness taste of or obesity genes and in addition the higher sugar resulted in more being burnt as fuel and consequently more fat storage. Another sleight of hand was to label low fat calories simply be providing reduced sizes. So while a low level of fat calories was consumed, the small portions required eating more portions for satiety resulting in fat calories over the desired amount. The end result is that while fat consumption has been reduced from 40% in 1990 to about 34% today, calorie consumed have gone up from 3,100 per capita per day in the 1960s to 3,700 in the 1990s per the US Department of Agriculture. That fact coupled with the decrease in activity in it does the math for the obesity epidemic.

d. Levels of Development

According to the World Health Organization [WHO] overweight and obesity is a function of a countries level of development with a few exceptions in special cases. Some of the factors of development and how they affect obesity are as follows.

Socioeconomic factors

In developed countries there is an inverse relationship between the prevalence of obesity and socioeconomic status. The rate of obesity certain groups in a high social class, is about one half as much as those of similar groups in the lower social classes. The exact reasons for this relationship have yet to be proven, but it has been repeatedly shown that overweight is a function of education, and it is a logical guess that the higher social classes are better educated. Associated with socioeconomic development in a developed country is the higher rate of competitiveness and increased pace of life. With this comes a higher level of stressful living, emotional suffering and there side effects of mental disorder, alcohol and drug abuse, violence, suicide and other behavioral problems, which have increased significantly in the last 3 decades, according to the World Health Organizations report of World Health 1998. Unnecessary eating and comforting one's self with fat and sweet foods has been shown to be associated with high stress and emotional suffering.

Rate of developmental growth - rapid economic growth of cultures almost always provide the increased opportunity to escape environment restraints and increase their consumption of energy dense foods and reduce activity. The move to the 'western' diet and lifestyles when the opportunity arises is almost universal.

Increasing Opportunity to eat - according to World Health Organization's World Health Report 1998, food supply has more than doubled in the past 40 years, much faster than population growth.

Spiritual - The rate of Hopelessness has increased as indicated to the decrease in religion in most of the developed countries. Religious growth has not grown in proportion to population increase and there is a decrease in morality

Inactivity - The level of activity has decreased due to labor saving devices and the way we earn our living.

Change in eating patterns and types of food - there have been a significant change in the departure from natural foods to processed food and eating patterns in developing countries. A significant change in eating patterns, including an increase in eating out, fast food and grazing. In a study published in *Obesity Research in 2002,* data taken from the Nationwide Food Consumption Survey for a sample of 63,380 of different age groups showed that the trends in eating patterns were essentially the same for all age groups, from the young to the old. The data showed the move away from meals at home to restaurants and from meals that required substantial preparation time to meals that were the quickest to prepare. The similar eating patterns and the increased calorie intake across all age groups show the obesity gene at work in a changes environment.

Educational

As a country becomes more developed, a high emphasis is placed on education and the higher its level of education the higher the motivation to improve health. A number of studies both in the US and in Europe showed that body weight was a function of education. This is also the case where studies show that in a given culture, the healthiest are usually the more educated, the assumption being that the more educated are more aware of the benefits of a healthy diet and exercise. This is not a big surprise, since with it is reasonable to think that when an individual is aware of the benefits of health they would do everything in their power to get as healthy as possible. However, it is obvious that education in itself is not sufficient to control the 'obesity genes'. Witness the highly educated religious communities in the US, the priests, nuns, ministers, etc. and their overwhelming level of obesity.

Other limitations of present levels of education and awareness are;

a. We are not educated in the disease risk factors of being overweight and obese-
b. We do not really believe in the pain resulting from overweight and obesity and the pleasure in being healthy
c. We are not in control of our minds when we eat [this is most likely true, since we are not usually not in control of our minds]
d. Our culture does not practice pleasure postponement for the greater good.
e. We are operating in a state of high stress.
f. We are not mindful of what we are eating, but rather thinking of something else, involved in conversations or reading that distracts our attention.

    g. Frequently the act of eating is more an emotional expression rather than a natural healthy physical need.

    h. The portions are too large and our culture teaches us to clean our plate.

e. Psychological

While Individuals may use strategies to minimize the risk of weight gain by the appropriate diet and exercise, the level of control that an individual is able to exert over their environment is not only influenced by the strength of their obesity genes and self-discipline, but also a number of psychological factors may come into play. As previously discussed, some people resort to overeating in response to distressing events or some other form of emotional suffering, while others find their appetite is reduced by such situations. What goes on in our heads frequently has a lot of influence on our eating habits. . Many studies show that people eat in response to negative emotions such as boredom, sadness, anxiety or anger. Studies have shown that higher than normal stress leads to the overproduction of the stress hormone cortisol, which boasts the appetite, Cortisol can be a part of a vicious circle of eating and stressing out, which can be a real problem since dieting is one of the most stressful things a person can do. Unhealthy programs of dieting can lead to a host of psychological and physiologically disorders.

    Emotional suffering- If we are emotionally uncomfortable and feel that are emotionally hungry we will turn to means of dealing our emotional discomfit [stress] and hopefully bring relief from our emotional pain. These potential satisfiers include alcohol, sex, physical activity, and food. Food being the most universal, socially acceptable and commonly available. While food [like the rest of these temporary comforters] may temporary numb our emotional suffering, and provide some degree of relief, it is short term at best. Since we haven't solved the under lying problem of emotional discomfort, the cycle will repeat itself.

    Lack of Mental control - Eastern Philosophies teaches that the prime cause of emotional suffering stems mainly from the inability to fulfill our desires. Our inability to use our mind to set realistic boundaries on our desires brings such suffering.

Lack of Self-esteem - Lack of love for coupled with a feeling of hopelessness, results in disrespect for our body and appearance

Low Energy – What is not well known, or at least difficult to believe, is that a gain in energy stems from physical activity. The more sedentary we are the more the less energy we will have. Low energy levels bring depression and a general reduction of the quality of life.

f. Food Consumerism

Like any profit orientated business's drive to sell more products at higher margins, our huge food industry's focus is to find ways to get people to eat as much high margin product as possible. This is the reality of what food consumerism is all about; the customer's health is not a bottom line concern. Consequently every opportunity that American inventiveness can conceive to entice us to consume more of their products is exploited. In addition we have a huge industry involved with TV and video games, with the same profit incentive, but in their case their focus is to get more eyes viewing their screens. The unhealthy combination of eating more while viewing more, provides more calories with less activity, a sure fire formula for weight gain. Intensifying this combination is the avenue to reinforce each other by promoting an association between food, fun, action figures, cartoons, spectator sports, etc. The reality is that the fatter and more inactive we are, the bigger their markets.

Marketing is aimed at children, who are equipped with the attention getting behavior that can motive the parents and the families food supply. Many studies show that the great majority of spontaneous food purchases are the result of a child demonstrating behavior difficult to ignore. In our American society, the family unit has one or two working parents living at a high pace of life and under high enough stress that leaves them too busy and stressed to study and enforce good nutrition. Desperate to keep the peace and please their children, they default to their off-spring's food desires. Due to the overabundance of food in the industrialized world, the concept of food marketing moves from healthy nourishment to image in hyping the young, more impressionable customers and effectively forming their food preferences and eating patterns.

Convenience and Fast Food

What started out as simple convenience, several decades ago, has turned the car into a substitute for the modern kitchen. The drive through window at the fast food emporium in now responsible of the majority of fast food sold in the US. Recent studies indicate that about one fourth of American adults eat fast food on any given day, and a significant number get fast food daily. Not that the drive through window is necessarily unhealthy, but that through its passes the poorest excuses for nutritious food imaginable. Without question, the rapid growth in fast food industry is a significant factor in replacing what little natural foods we do eat with high energy fat, sweet and processed food. We now eat our potatoes as hydrogenated vegetable oil soaked, chips, French fries and hash browns. And by itself, fast food is basically responsible for the huge increase in our consumption of cheese; in cheese foods and melted onto burgers, pizza, pasta and nachos. To keep an even playing field, we have provided the rest of the world with our fast food expertise, and they have generally embraced the opportunity to transcend their culture and become as fat as we are.

Convenience with taste is what fast food is all about, and consequently much of the advertising is focused on how we don't have the time to shop, prepare and mindfully eat our meals. And the convenience angle has taken its toll, reducing typical dinner preparation time from over 2 hours to less than 15 minutes in the past few decades, aided by the technology that has made this possible. In these days' it's hard to image any home with working parents without a microwave and frozen foods, and more recently this has even extended to retired seniors. Uncontrolled food consumerism may well be the main cause our 'obesity genes' are in control. The continuous barrage of hype from the food producer and leisure industry beats down our defenses, and gives us an easy way out to satisfy our children and eliminate taking the time to plan and/or prepare healthy meals. And while Federal agencies publish healthy food guidelines, our Federal Agencies are influenced by the industries that they are unable/unwilling to control. On one hand, it can be said that the expansion of these industries and their job generating and tax producing benefits are in the tradition of American business, it can also be said that profit generation at the cost of the detraction the health of our citizens is a cost far in excess of the benefits. As a comparison, the benefits and human costs of the tobacco industry comes to mind.

Value Marketing-or how to get fatter cheaper.

The factor of food consumerism that seems to appeal to the majority is to get more calories for less money. According to a health newsletter from Tufts University, it's not just restaurant meals that are getting bigger, even diet foods have swelled to 'hearty portion' sizes that weight up to 50 percent more than the original. Even some the better known weight loss programs are advertising larger portions, and the trend is insidious. Even car manufacturers installing larger cup holders to fit the ever-increasing size of fast food beverages to go with their swelling size of super burgers and fries which have tripled in size since about 1960. Unfortunately, in today's environment, a substantial number of studies substantiate that people whether they are men or women, normal or overweight, dieting or unrestrained eaters take portions larger then they need. There is much truth in the well-known saying that people eat with their eyes instead of their stomach.

A recent article in American Institute for Cancer Research newsletter, entitled "Value Marketing is Making Americans Fat" started out by stating that foreign visitors to this country always comment on two things: the portion sizes in our restaurants are huge, and too many Americans are overweight. This certainly comes as no surprise to most of us. Personally, I have heard it from foreign visitors many times. I also found the reverse to be generally true when traveling overseas. When visiting Paris France some 30 years ago, and again recently, I was amazed at two things, [besides the traffic and the Louve] the small portions served at the restaurants [and also the homes of friends], and the comparative thinnest of the French compared to Americans. It doesn't take a great stretch to believe that the low calorie intake of the French is responsible for at least part of the reason for the 'French Paradox' [relatively high fat diet with a relatively low incidence of heart disease].

The underlying concept of value marketing has to do with selling people more of something for less than a proportional increase in money. For instance, getting a 2 pounder for just a little more money than a one pounder. It makes economic sense for the food industry because you can give customers value either by cutting prices or putting more food on the plate. When it comes to a choice between cutting prices by a dollar or giving people about thirty cents extra food, it's not a difficult choice. While this may sound attractive to some, the problem is that it doesn't take much extra food, on a regular basis, to make a substantial difference in body weight. The U.S. Department of Agriculture [USDA] figures show that just eating an additional 148 calories per day on average could work out to an extra 15 pounds per year.

Two new studies published in the Journal of the American Medical Association and the Journal of the American Dietetic Association; tell us we are simply eating more of the same foods than we did 20 years because portion sizes have increased. Portion sizes for most foods served in the home and at a restaurants have increased so that we consume 93 calories more in a serving of salty snacks, 49 more in soft drinks, 50 more in fruit drinks, 97 more in hamburgers and 133 more from Mexican food.

One of the shifts in American society that may have had a significant impact on our collective weight is the acceptance of eating in public places. Shopping malls, book stores, movies, grocery stores, sports stadiums, fitness studios, etc. all offer drink and snack bars [unlikely to have health food]. Half the food ordered at fast food restaurants is now through the drive-up window, and commonly people eat in their cars. Needless to say, snacks on the run usually are not planned and turn out as excess unhealthy calories. This behavior of eating whenever, wherever, and whatever, undoubtedly plays a significant part in our collective overweight.

Medical disorders

Very few individuals have a medical condition which increases the likelihood of becoming obese. Hypothyroidism leads to a reduction in resting metabolic rate and Cushing's syndrome promotes fat deposition. Abnormalities of other hormones can affect body weight and fat distribution. However appropriate treatment usually eliminates the problem. Also certain drugs can lead to changes in body weight or fat distribution. Corticosteroids and some antidepressant and antihistamine drugs can stimulate appetite, increasing energy intake and promoting fat storage around the midsection, if taken long enough. However, the above are estimated to be responsible for only about 1 percent of all obesity

CHAPTER THREE

Why weight loss programs
can be weight gain programs

1. Background
2. Popular trends in current diets
3. The yo-yo effect
4. Weight loss drugs are not the answer
5. About carbohydrates
6. Major types of diets
7. Why popular diets can't work?
8. Why the OGD does work

1. Background

As previously stated, the National Institutes of Health has shown that the majority of currently popular weight loss programs fail within one year and 95% fail within five years. The formula of the diet makes little difference. No matter the combination of macronutrients; whether they are high or low fat, carbs, or proteins, or any combination thereof makes little difference with regard to long term weight loss. And adding special foods, be it sugar, grapefruit, or whatever, doesn't improve the success. The few programs that do have some limited weight loss success involve continuous support and hand holding. The biological facts and physics involved

53

in weight loss are based on calories rather than food type. Calorie intake [actually absorbed] less calories burnt [resting plus active] is the fundamental equation for weight change. Second order effects, such as differences in metabolic rate, absorption, chemical imbalances, and other mechanisms that effect the energy formula, causes losses that can explain why some people can seemingly eat more than others without gaining weight. More recently, some studies indicate that genetics may play a hand in this. Consequently, no matter how the promoter attempts to claim a unique combination of micronutrients [fats, carbs or protein] or eating patterns, the reality is that calories are calories.

To lose weight, it is necessary to eat fewer calories and/or to burn more. As previously discussed, while this sounds simple to the uninformed, it is fact not realistic due to the urgings of our obesity genes and unhealthy eating habits. In addition, most trendy diets are unproven and ignore the science of nutrition and the healthy success of the HALL peoples. Based on defective science, and opinions, these diet programs are profit motivated [or at best misguided] to take advantage of an unknowledgeable public for a program that can't work and may be harmful.

However, despite all the warning of healthcare organizations and Government programs, the unpleasant reality is that the over $40 billion spent in the escalating weight loss market, is not having any positive effect on the souring weight gain of Americans. You might even say that popular diet plans actually cause weight gain, since their false promises distract dieters from seeking effective methods of weight reduction.

2. Popular trends in current diets

There are over 50 million adult Americans presently on some kind of a diet, and they have more weight loss programs to choose from than any other people. Consumers are inundated with choices as each provider attempts to uniquely distance itself, using such terms as: "New Revolutionary Approach", 'Eat your way to dynamic weight loss', 'Finally, an easy way to lose weight, 'Weight loss breakthroughs', and a host of celebrity, and beautiful people diets. With all the conflicting claims and promises, the uninformed consumer is understandably left in a state of confusion. Added to this confusion, is the reality that there are no credible long term clinical trials to provide scientific substantiation for any of the popular diet programs.

In addition, as we are all biologically unique and have different needs for types and quantities of calories. Your calorie requirements to achieve a desired goal, depends on many different factors, including activity level, gender, age, height, present weight and body frame. You can calculate a rough estimate of your calories needs to maintain your weight by multiplying your weight by 10 for females and 11 for males. This is the approximate amount of calories is required for your resting metabolism, to which should be added the calories required for you for your physical activities. However, since we don't really think of ourselves so scientifically as biological machines, this type of thinking gets ignored by the average person concerned with weight loss. At any rate, for the normal situation, the goal is to eventually get to a healthy weight as determined by your Body Mass Index, as discussed in Chapter One.

Because the diet field is unscientific and not regulated, it is wide open to exploitation by any opportunist that knows how to sell. Providers are virtually free to make any claim [except a disease cure] they think will sell the program, book, product, service, etc. In lieu of scientific proof, they attempt to support their claims by testimonials, antidotal stories, and other types of junk science. In addition most of the current programs are nothing more than recycled old strategies dressed up in new packages, as though they were new discoveries. The National Institutes of Health, free from the incentive of the profit motive, provides a scientific approach to a healthy diet and guidelines to weight loss. Unfortunately, even these diet programs have the same shortcoming as the rest, in that they don't provide behavioral change programs required to change eating habits.

3. The yo-yo effect

One of the most common threats to health from discretionary diet-ing, is the so called 'yo-yo' effect, where the dieters weight goes down and up with their eating patterns like a yo-yo. As discussed in the last chapter, the body's internal set point mechanism for regu-lation of body fat acts to maintain an amount of body fat within cer-tain norms. When you diet and lose weight once, the body senses that famine has struck and it learns from the experience. The next time you diet the body rapidly compensates for the lost calories by reducing your metabolic rate, thereby reducing the effect of calo-rie restriction. As a result, depending on the relative amounts of calories and rate of metabolism, your weight can actually increase, even though you are eating comparative fewer calories, creating the yo-yo effect which is eventually self-defeating as well as dangerous. Repeated yo-yo dieting has been associated with increased heart disease in the Framingham health study. All diets that result in at least initial weight loss, by definition, must involve reducing your normal intake of calories. A diet motivated by will power, that just uses the innovation of reducing calories, regardless of macronutri-ent combinations, is predestined to failure the influence of 'obesity genes'. It has been estimated that less than 5% of people have the tremendous discipline to substantially reduce calorie intake for any extended time. Your body soon gets your attention with excruciat-ing hunger pangs, headaches, lack of energy and any other physical and emotional pain it can bring to bear. The deprivation type of diet program has been attempted forever, with a seemingly unlim-ited variety of wrinkles, but the results are always the same. The reality is that people can't handle hunger when there is a choice.

4. Weight loss drugs are not the answer

Many researchers are convinced that effective drug treatments are imminent and obesity, just like hypertension and diabetes will soon be treated with pills, but this is typical American medicine mentality. As is common knowledge, all pills interfere with our biological systems, resulting in some kind of side effects. And side effects can result in a host of unhealthy effects that can be individualistic and not infrequently show up later as a serious problem. In a race to produce profits before safety and efficacy is proven, the history of diet drugs is littered with famous failures, and here are the most significant...

Leptin - In a search for the gene that controls hunger, gene researchers experimenting with mice came to the conclusion that leptin seems to be the long sought satiety factor. The breakthrough was thought to come in 1994, with the discovery of leptin, a protein that obese mice lacked. Giving the protein to obese mice made them thin and Amgen a California biotechnology company paid millions for the right to develop a weight loss drug. But studies proved disappointing. Few peoples have leptin deficiencies and giving leptin to most others did nothing to help them lose pounds...

Fen-pen - Then came the fen-phen fiasco, with its disastrous side effects. In 1984 fen-phen was promoted as a powerful weighs loss agent after a four year study show that, on average, women taking the drug lost 6 pounds more than did women taking a placebo, however, little was known of long term side effects. In spite of its limited success, it was marketed by just about everyone in the business, from Jenny Craig, to Readers Digest. Then the lack of doing the due diligence clinical testing caught up with them and serious side effects emerged. In 1994, the cases of congestive heart failure and other serious side effects, including a couple of deaths, and over 4,000 suits had been filed making it one of the largest product liability cases in history.

Redux - In the 1970 a French pharmaceutical company developed a technique to produce pure dexfenfluarmine, a component of fen phen, which it branded Redux. In spite of a significant list of side effects, Redux, in 1996, became the first diet drug in more than twenty years to gain FDA approval and had the history of a shooting star. Shooting up and then plunging down.

Meridia - when Meridia entered the U.S. market, sales of the drug soared to more than $108 million in 1998 but sales slipped the following year. A massive ad campaign failed to resuscitate sales which continued to plummet on increasing news that few people who took Meridia lost weight and some even gained.

Xenical- the FDA approved this diet aid in 1999 and it is presently the best selling prescription weight loss drug on the market. Xenical acts in the chemistry of the gut rather than the central nervous system, as do previous weight loss drugs and consequently doctors feel more comfortable in prescribing it. Taking Xenical before a meal causes about one third of fat eaten to pass through the intestine undigested. Known side effects include passing oily gas and increased and uncontrollable bowel movements, which gives a strong incentive to reduce fat consumption. The nominal benefits are said to be a nominal weight loss in six months that returns in about 2 years. Long term side effects are unknown.

Ephedra - a Chinese herbal remedy used for several thousand years is the best known weight loss aid in the diet field. As an herbal supplement it is not regulated by the FDA and can be marketed anywhere by anyone. Its active ingredient Ephedrine is used in a variety of weight loss products, the best known being Metabolife There is currently a lot of bad press on ephedra associated side effects, including hypertension, stroke, seizures and tachycardia, being published in prestigious medical journals. Scientific studies of its safety and efficacy are not available – buyers beware. Ephedra was recently banned by the FDA in early 2004, and is being removed from various products on the market

Ghrelin - Today, the hottest research focuses on the natural hormone ghrelin, first identified by Japanese scientist in 1999. Ghrelin seems to increase appetite. Scientists at the University of Washington recently found that dieters who lose weight produce extra ghrelin, which could be why they become ravenous and regained every very lost pound. Ghrelin could drive eating too according to some scientists and they are trying to unravel how the hormone works in hopes of devising a pill that will safely curb hunger. At this point, there is a very long way to reach safety and efficacy standards

The questionable efficacy of weight loss drugs

Weight loss drugs are another case of man manipulating nature, and consequently have an uncertain future. The complex biological design of food intake and processing by the nature of its survival value, is very complex with backup protection, and fail safe systems which resist reengineering. Consequently it seems unlikely to fool Mother Nature with our present level of biological knowledge. All the more reason for finding a natural way to satisfy our 'obesity genes' in a way that allows a healthy weight loss.

5. About carbohydrates

There is much misunderstanding about carbohydrates [carbs], as evidenced by the current craze on low carb foods. To make it simpler to discuss, consider two kinds of carbs, complex-the good carb and simple – the bad carb. First let's talk about the good carb. Since it supplies the majority of the OGD eating program. The high complex carbohydrates diet [plant based] is recommended by the NIH, WHO, most health authorities, and is the natural diet of the world's HALL peoples, described in chapter 4. While there are various nuances, the foundation of the diet is complex carbohydrates. Complex carbs are specified, since in the days of long lived peoples, that is basically the only type available, while today, the market is proliferated with processed simple carbohydrates. Complex carbohydrates are the majority of our natural diet, the diet of our ancestors that still suits our genetic programming. In essence, plant foods are packages of water, held together by fiber. Since water contains no calories and fiber only minute amounts, plant foods fill you up without adding significant weight. For instance, a large tomato of the same weight as lean ground beef has less than a tenth of calories. The sheer volume of food in a plant based meal will stretch your stomach receptors to signal your brain that you are full.

Carbohydrates are composed from the chemical components, carbon, oxygen and hydrogen. Variation of their chemical structure results in the two basic forms of carbohydrates, simple carbs,

-the 'bad' carb [table sugar, cakes, white bread] and complex carbs- the 'good' carb. [I.e. Natural plant foods, such as fruits, vegetables and whole grains,] The simple, or bad carbs have been refined [fiber removed i.e. bleached white flour] while the complex or good carbs are unrefined [fiber present - whole grain flours, fruit and beans] the unrefined complex carbs contain most of their natural vitamins, minerals and other antioxidants. The indigestible fiber of the complex carb slows the absorption while when the fiber is stripped away, the simple carbohydrates get absorbed quicker.

Some of the bad press for carbs stems from misinterpretation of the Glycemic Index [GI]. In simple terms, the Glycemic Index is a means that indicates the amount blood sugar rises after eating a particular carbohydrate. Carbs that break down the fastest, raise blood sugar the most. The index is related to pure glucose, such that a GI of 80 would have 80% of the effect of pure glucose. Since the amount of blood sugar [glucose] in our blood stream is regulated by insulin, the pancreas releases insulin to take glucose from the blood stream and pack it into cells. When you eat quick release, simple carbohydrate food, like cookies, white bread and cake the glucose rises rapidly in the blood stream and as a consequence, increased insulin is produced to eliminate the excess glucose. Since the glucose-insulin is not synced perfectly, in the process of reducing the glucose, theory is some overshoot and your blood sugar level will drop low. The result is that with a meal high in simple carbs and particularly high GI, your glucose will spike, which increases insulin and fat storage. In comparison, eating slow release low GI foods such whole grain bread, high fiber fruits and vegetables, the glucose in your blood stream increases slower and to a less degree, causing the pancreas to producer much smaller amounts of insulin. This is a good thing, because causing the pancreas to correct high swings in glucose, over time, is a risk factor for diabetes. Keeping the blood sugar levels moderate over a longer period of time, you feel less hungry less often. Smaller meals also have s similar effect and actually allow us to nibble more often without gaining fat.

6. Major types of diets

The low carb craze

Since this marketing trend does not discern between 'good' and 'bad' carbs, the public has been misled, suggesting that the promotion frenzy on 'low carb' is all about making money. All kinds of food products have been reengineered, repacked, renamed and whatever other scheme will sell the public on the present low carb craze. While it's true that reduced simple or refined carbs [white bread, cakes, cookies, etc.] are good candidates for weight loss, it is just the opposite with complex carbs. [Natural plant foods]. Presenting the difference between the good or natural carb and the bad or refined carb would give the public healthy nutrition advice. But this likely won't be done for the simple reason that you can't make the profit margins on natural foods that you can when you can pass along the processing and refining costs. Consequently, the marketing hype is directed on scaring people away from all carbs, 'good' and 'bad'.

High Protein Diets

In the recent past, the American public has been confused by best-selling books which claim that high-carbohydrate eating programs *cause* weight gain and that low carbohydrate, high protein; high fat [Atkins] diets cause people to lose weight. As mentioned above, little distinction is made between complex and simple forms of carbs. The bottom line is that high protein diets haven't been proven to work in the long-term and, according to the National Institutes of Health and other reputable sources, due to the high level of saturated and trans-fat involved, they are prescriptions for early heart attacks. "Individuals who follow these diets are at risk for compromised vitamin and mineral intake, as well as potential cardiac, renal, bone, and liver abnormalities overall," according to the American Heart Association Journal *Circulation.* Recently a randomized trial of a low carbohydrate, high protein, high-fat [Atkins] diet was conducted to evaluate its efficacy, and reported in the New England Journal of Medicine. A one year controlled trial involving 63 obese men and women were randomly assigned to the Atkins diet or a low calorie, high carbohydrate, low fat [conventional] diet. The conclusion were that the low-carbohydrate diet produced a greater weight loss of about 4 percent than did the conventional for the first six months, but the differences were not significant at one year. The low carbohydrate diet was associated with a greater improvement in some risk factors for coronary heart disease. Adherence was poor and attrition was high in both groups. Recently, the Atkins diet has fallen into disfavor and its diet business discontinued, due to lack of long term success and the demise of its overweight founder.

Noted food researchers have examined the diets of virtually all healthier countries and found that almost all ingest less animal-based protein, and more complex carbohydrates than we do in the US. Virtually all noted nutrition researchers advise us to eat a greater proportion of our calories as complex carbohydrate-rich whole grains, vegetables and fruits and ingest a smaller proportion of calories from refined sugar products, high-protein/high fat meats, and dairy products. Unfortunately, currently popular conventional high-carbohydrate diets in the US. And other westernized countries don't work for many people either. Many contain too many simple carbohydrates, the type of carbohydrate that rapidly breaks down into glucose (sugar) causing our blood sugars and then our insulin levels to spike. Even the very low fat and high complex carbohydrate programs are not practical for most people long term because they are too demanding and require foods that lack the taste and satisfaction desired by most Americans. People start craving the taste of fat and simple, sugar-based carbohydrates and then "fall off" those unbalanced programs because they have not learned how to retrain their ingrained former eating habits.

As a result, they often regain not only the weight they lost but even more, causing 'yo-yo' dieting which can put them at higher risk of debilitating diseases.

High protein diets [mostly animal foods] and low carbs are currently trendy for the uninformed person seeking only quick results. And admittedly for good reason, since they reduce calories, they frequently produce initial weight loss. For obvious reasons, the popularity of the high protein diet stems mainly from those who normally have high total fat diet habits and are encouraged by the initial weight loss. It seems to them almost too good to be true, that you can eat all the animal fat that you want, eliminate the less palatable fruits and vegetables and still lose weight. And not much later, you find out that indeed it is too good to be true as the weight soon returns. In addition, if you are on this diet for any significant period you have likely increased your risk factors for heart disease, stroke and cancer.

The promoters claim that it induces a state called ketosis is which appetite is suppressed and initially water is shed causing weight loss. The diet reduces hunger so you eat fewer calories and lose more weight. According to an article in *the Tufts University Health and Nutrition Letter: June 2002,* food researchers have shown that virtually all countries recommend less protein and more carbohydrate, and advise to eat a greater proportion of calories as carbohydrate-rich grains, vegetables and fruits and a smaller proportion as high-protein meat and dairy. Researchers at the University of Illinois highlighted the universality of recommendations when they systematically reviewed the nutrition guide pictorials of 12 countries around the globe. While there were differences in smaller details, due to cultural preferences, each country's basic recommendation was to get the bulk of calories from complex carbohydrates and fewer from protein rich foods [which are often are rich in saturated fat as well]. Of still greater significance is the fact that none of the HALL long lived peoples, have high protein diets, but instead, get the majority of their calories from complex carbohydrate diets. In addition, countries with the lowest incidence of the degenerative diseases such as heart and cancer eat mainly natural plant based diets.

While the fact is high protein diets have been periodically popular since the 1960's, there still is no scientific studies or even credible supporting evidence to indicate their effectiveness on weight loss and safety. According to a study in the American Heart Association Journal Circulation, *2001; 104; 1869-1874* "Individuals who follow these diets are at risk for compromised vitamin and mineral intake, as well as potential cardiac, renal, bone, and liver abnormalities overall" High Protein diets typically offer wide latitude in protein food choices, but generally are high in total fat, saturated fat, and cholesterol since the protein is usually from animal sources. The promoters of these diets, lacking any scientific evidence of their efficacy and safety, resort to defective claims concerning insulin resistance, ketosis and carbohydrates, and fat burning. Contrary to claims the initial weight loss is initially high due to fluid loss related to reduced carbohydrate intake, overall calorie restriction and ketosis-induced appetite suppression. Further, any effects on blood lipids and insulin resistance are due to weight loss, rather than carbohydrate restriction.

The sellers of a high protein, low carbohydrate diets claim that by restricting carbohydrates to a mere fraction of that recommended by health authorities, the body goes into a state of ketosis, where it burns its own fat for fuel. When the body is in ketosis you tend to feel less hungry and consequently eat less than you might otherwise. However ketosis can also cause a variety of unpleasant effects. When your body changes from a carbo-burning engine into fat-burning engine, your fat stores become a primary energy source and the purported result is weight loss. Another selling feature for low carbohydrates is that on a high carbohydrate diet, sugar from the carbohydrates quickly enters the bloodstream, and to keep it from rising too high, the body secretes insulin. Insulin then allows the extra sugar to eventually be stored into fat. With eating too much sugar, we may become less responsive to insulin and develop a metabolic disorder, which leads to the early stages of diabetes, but a body ketosis burn up excess fat in time return to normal metabolic function. While there is some truth in this, it is only the case when the carbohydrates in question are simple, like sugar, rather than complex carbohydrates, such as plant foods. . However insulin secretion is also effected by a number of interacting factors such as obesity and lack of physical activity and can be lowered by caloric restriction, weight loss and exercise But in any event, there is no disagreement form either side of the controversy that high levels of sugar intake is to be avoided.

The promoters of high-protein, low-carbohydrate diets claim that high-carbohydrate diets raise the blood level of insulin and that insulin causes weight gain by storing food in fat cells. This has been proven untrue by a recent study. According to Tufts University *Health & Nutrition* July 2003, researchers at Michigan State and Harvard compared the insulin levels of almost 12,000 men and women to the number of calories they ate as carbohydrates. Those who's carbohydrate intake was 60 percent or higher, had no higher levels of insulin than those who's intake was 40 percent or less. According to researchers, insulin doesn't route food to fat cells, only eating more calories than you burn does that.

According to a summary of a study the American Heart Association Science Advisory, there are no scientific studies that show that high protein diets, without less caloric intake result in long term weigh loss or improved health. Most Americans consume more protein needed and extra protein is not used efficiently by the body and may impose a metabolic burden on the kidneys and liver. Most importantly, there is a wealth of credible studies and clinical tests well published by health agencies indicating that high fat diets are a major risk factor for heart disease, strokes and some forms of cancer. and last, but not least, countries with the highest animal fat intake have the highest level of degenerative diseases and the shortest life span, [some examples are; Scotland, Germany, Finland, Great Britain, etc.] while countries with the lowest animal fat intake have the lowest level of degenerative diseases and longest life spans [some examples are tradition diets of Mediterranean, Japan, Rural China, Okinawa, etc.] Various media articles reported that a physician group, critical of the Atkins diets stated that Dr. Atkins, creator of the high-protein, low-carb "Atkins Diet", may have had heart disease when he died at age 72, after slipping on an icy street and hitting his head. According to an article in the Wall Street Journal on 11 Feb the medical examiner's report noted that Atkins had a history of heart trouble, including congestive heart failure and high blood pressure, In April 2002, Atkins issued a statement saying he was recovering from cardiac arrest relating to a heart infection he had suffered from "for a few years" He said it was "in no way related to his diet" Whether or not his poor health was related to the Atkins Diet, is a matter of conjecture, however even his supporters agree he weighed 195 pounds before entering the hospital. At 6 ft., this puts his BMI at 26.4, which is in the overweight category, and hardly the ideal figure head of a healthy diet.

Very low-fat, High Carbohydrate Diets

There are a number of high carbohydrates diets on the market in addition to the ones published by the major world health agencies that specify very low fats. [I.e. 10% or less] The degree and special preferences put some originality on some of these, but the basic principles are the same, but aside from this they all have the same basic principles of maximizing natural plant foods and minimizing saturated fat and processed foods, accompanied by physical activity. One of best known diets largely based on vegetables, grains and fruits get close to a vegetarian diet with keeping fat portions down in the 10% area. More recent enhancements focus on calorie density. By filling up on foods that are not calorie dense, you have the freedom to eat until you are full without calorie counting and food restriction. The basic plan is to eat food with a large volume of fiber and water, such as vegetables, fruits, beans and natural unprocessed grains in order not to fill hungry or deprived, or have need to count calories. This reduces the intake of processed the foods are more likely to be calorie dense compared to natural foods. For instance, corn starts out in its natural state at about 490 calories per pound, and increases to about 2,400 calories when it becomes a pound of tortilla chips. One of these plans use a guideline of keeping the average caloric density of each meal below 400 calories per pound. Vegetables usually are below 200 calories per pound, and high carbohydrate meals range between 230 to 630 calories per pound while animal protein ranges from 400 to 1,400 calories per pound. While these types of diets have gone beyond the typical HALL diets and they are difficult to adjust to and many will find them deprived of the palatable taste of fat and difficult to follow, since they are contra to our subconscious program for fat.

Other very low fat high carbs programs claim that eating a high-fiber, low-fat vegetarian diet will not only will help you lose weight but will also help you stay healthy. The types of foods you eat are of prime interest, rather than restricting calories. Unlimited Vegetables, Fruits, Whole grains, grains and legumes can be eaten, until full. Foods eaten in moderation include nonfat dairy products, [skim mile nonfat yogurt and cheese and egg whites]. Foods to be avoided include; animal meat of all kinds, [including fish], oils avocados, olives, nuts and seeds, dairy products, sugar and derivatives, alcohol, any processed food with more the two grams of fat per serving.

This plan provides less than 10% of calories from fat. It is generally recommended that eating a number of little meals [at the minimum 3 meals with 2 snacks] will help you feel full on fewer calories. As with other similar types of diets, exercise and stress management are required. This routine avoids the body's ability to decrease the rate of metabolism that comes with calorie restriction. The idea is to eat sufficiently to avoid feeling starved and having our genetic program reduce our metabolism. Some of these programs also use meditation to increase self-awareness and reduce stress. While these types of programs are close to the diets of the healthiest and long lived, except for their restriction go good fats, such as fish and nuts and olive oil. Another popular diet type is similar to that of the traditional Mediterranean countries.

traditional meaning up to about 1960. After that time, the Medi-terranean countries became more and more Westernized is diet and lifestyles, becoming more animal oriented and less plant ori-ented. Their laudable low level of obesity and heart disease, have been catching up with the Western countries since then. The diet component about 50 to 60% of the calories in carbohydrates, with as much as possible as complex from unrefined grains and vegeta-bles that release glucose into the bloodstream more slowly. Fats are up to 30% of the calories with most being monounsaturated oils, such as olive oil and foods high in omega-3 fatty acids, such as fatty fish, flax seeds and walnuts. Protein should be limited to 10-20% of your diet using vegetable proteins, such as beans and soybean, with as little animal protein as possible.

Have we been led astray by our Government?

We have also been given bad advice from the US government and the nation's largest and most respected health organizations. For decades Americans were told the primary cause of weight gain was eating fatty, greasy goods. A healthy diet was heavy in carbo-hydrates, such as bread, cereals, and pasta that formed the wide base of the government's highly touted food pyramid. Fruits and vegetables come next. then meat and dairy. Americans have taken this nutrition advice. We eat much less dietary fat now than we did the 1950s. But our national lower fat, high- carbohydrate diet has been a miserable failure in the fight against obesity. The problem lies in the type; of carbohydrates consumed.

The typical 'American diet is high in refined carbohydrates such a white bread, white rice, pasta and potatoes as opposed to unprocessed carbohydrates such as whole grains. The major problem with the refined carbohydrates is that they are quickly digested and send natural sugar [glucose] into your blood stream. This causes your pancreas to release insulin and absorb the sugar resulting in a sudden drop in glucose which can make you hun-gry again. Some physicians believe these rapid spikes or fluctua-tions in blood sugar are a significant cause of obesity. These rapid swings up and down in blood sugar do stimulate the appetite and make it harder for some people to control what they eat and lose weight. Meanwhile the physicians are not about to recommend the trendy high fat high protein diet to obese Americans. They know that most all diets work at first, because they force people to focus of what they eat, [or rather how much they eat] and many initially lose weight.

In addition to a faulty food pyramid [the most recent pyramid has been improved], it is assumed that people with sufficient will power can follow them. But as the concept of the obesity cause shows, that is not the case. This is not to assume that only Americans have little willpower, most all other cultures fit the same mold. That's why doctors, until recently, regarded obesity as primarily a psychological problem, one brought on a lack of willpower. Today scientists know that the problem is as much if not more physical in nature. What molecular biology has told us over the past decade is that there is a very complex regulating system that controls the body weight... More than 40 genes are likely to play a role in determining how much fat and muscle you carry on your frame.

The US initiative on eating low fat foods may have had some success on reducing risks for heart disease, but overweight continues its spiral upward. While it's true that fat has about twice the calories per gram as protein and carbohydrates and if we just ate equal grams of food a new diet with less fat would contain fewer calories. While this works in theory, it is usually impractical since we are likely to initially eat more calories on a low fat diet, because it is initially less hunger satisfying. Another complicating fact is the difference between simple and complex carbohydrates. While low fat usually translates to more carbohydrates, if simple carbohydrates are prioritized, the effect can be to raise insulin levels that rev up the appetite. These issues are part of the complexity of the obesity pandemic but they are only peripheral to root cause of the 'obesity genes' unrestrained by a changed environment.

7. Why popular diets can't work.

o Excessive hunger is the undoing of virtual every calorie restrictive weight-loss program, because hunger goes against your genetic code which emotionally punishes by discomfort and pain.

o Hunger and the desire for fat defeat 95% of portion-control dieters.

o Any program that requires you to avoid plant foods is lacking in the nutrition necessary to reduce the risk factor of the major diseases.

o It is difficult to really believe in them since they are not based on proven success,

o They do not provide some method of mind conditioning to epigenetically modify our 'obesity genes'

o For a practical program, you must be able to eat until you reach fullness or satiety and eat whenever you are hungry. .

o You must enjoy the diet. Since food is one of our greatest pleasures, this need for satisfaction must be met.

o Our instinctive need for fat and sweets must be fulfilled

o The diet must be practical in that it can be enjoyed in virtually any environment.

o The program must include a practical program of exercise.

o There must be a supportive method to help the individual form healthy eating and exercise habits.

o They don't treat the whole person, body mind and spirit.

o Some are based on unhealthy diets that are risk factors for heart disease, stroke, cancer and diabetes

o Are based on unproven principles and personal opinions.

o Use a one size fits all approach, regardless of personal differences

o Do not support the habit development required for long term changes

o Market initial weight loss and disregard long term success.

o Are marketed using personalities, testimonies and other unscientific hype
o Can't be done from any location on an interactive basis.
o Most weight loss plans are based on deprivation; counting calories, restricting portion sizes and eating less food. Sooner or later, people get tired of feeling hungry, so they get off the diet, regain the weight and blame them self for not having enough discipline or motivation
o Don't provide practical exercise programs for different abilities
o Allow too much opportunistic eating

8. Why the Obesity Genes Diet [OGD] works

The top seven reasons why the OGD can help you lose weight NOW and keep it off the rest of your life!

o The OGD is the only scientifically based diet that includes epigenetic signals to modify subconscious programming for overeating.
o The OGD allows you to eat until you reach fullness or satiety and eat whenever you are hungry.
o The OGD will allow you to enjoy your food. Since food is one of our greatest pleasures, this need for satisfaction must be met.
o The OGD will allow you to satisfy your genetic need for fat and sweets.
o The OGD is the most practical eating plan in the market today and can be enjoyed in your home, at work, or even on vacation.
o The OGD provides practical exercise programs for different abilities that can be done in just a few minutes a day.

CHAPTER FOUR

The worlds healthiest and
longest lived [HALL] peoples

The Elder Okinawans
Traditional rural Chinese
Traditional Mediterranean Countries

The Elder Okinawans

Okinawans, who were born before the World War II period, lived on a diet mainly from the local plant foods and marine life, which involved considerable physical activity to bring the food to the table. Their predominant plant food diet, high activity and stress free life styles produced the world's healthiest and longest lived peoples according to the 25 year Okinawa Centenarian Study. This plant based diet and high physical activity and continues today for those Okinawans' termed the 'elders', as does their very low level of degenerative diseases, compared with Western countries. For example, heart disease is about 80% less than in the US and the incidence of cardiovascular diseases and cancer is the lowest in the world. Their centenarians are about 6 times as great as the US, with many of them still living independently.

The elder Okinawans are lean with an average body mass index of 20, while in the U.S. a comparative body mass index is about 25.8. The elder Okinawans stay lean not only by eating a low calorie, unrefined complex carbohydrate diet, but also have a habit of backing away from the table when they feel about 80% full. Although they probably didn't know the biological reasons behind this habit, the fact is that our stomach stretch receptors don't signal the brain until about 20 minutes after we eat. Consequently, if we eat until we feel full, about 20 minutes later we will feel stuffed and uncomfortable. In addition, overeating stretches the stomach, stimulating eating more the next time with the process continuing and requiring more and more food. Physical activity is a way of life, not only in manual labor, but also in leisure time activities, such as yoga, traditional dances, the martial arts, walking, gardening, etc.

The Okinawan elders diet is about 80% plant food and consists of the following

Mostly natural unprocessed foods	Servings	Frequency
Vegetables of wide variety	7 - 13	Per day
Grains- mostly whole - bread, rice, noodles, cereals	7 - 13	Per day
Fruit	2-4	Per day
Flavonoid Foods [i.e. - soy flakes, flaxseed, miso, tea]	2-4	Per day
Calcium Foods - [i.e. -skim milk, green leafy vegetables, soy milk and beans]	2-4	Per day
Omega -3 Foods [i.e.-fatty fish, flaxseed]	1-3	Per day
Vegetable Oils	1-2 tbls	Per day
Tea [i.e.- black, green, oolong]	1-3	Daily
Minimize - Optional		
Meat, Poultry and eggs	0-5	Per Week
Sweets	0-3	Per Week

Note – serving sizes are smaller than US size
In addition to this diet, the elder Okinawans follow the following eating principles

1. They believe that less is best, serve portions about 1/2 US size and leave the table with a slight hunger.

2. They eat a wide variety of foods [at least 15],

3. Eat mindfully and are aware of the full pleasure of the eating experience.

4. Eat slowly to prevent overeating, and properly chew food for good digestion.

5. Believe that lean is healthy and overweight is not.

6. Eat natural carbohydrates and high fiber foods to help keep calories low without a feeling of starvation. A sort of a 'eat more weigh less' strategy.

Comparison with US diets - as a percent of diet

Food	US	Okinawan	Okinawan sources
Vegetables	16	34	Raw, cooked and juices
Fruits	20	6	Raw, cooked, juices
Flavonoid rich	1	12	Beans, flaxseed, legumes, soy
Grains	11	32	Whole grains, bread, cereals, rice
Omega 3	1	11	Fish, olive oil, nuts, flaxseed
Meat/poultry/ eggs	29	3	
Calcium rich	22	2	Dairy, seaweed

Lifestyles of the Elder Okinawans

7. High coping skills and an optimistic attitude

8. Strong family ties and social networks,

9. Physical activity is a way of life, when not involved in manual labor they practice the martial arts and celebrate with traditional dancing

10. Their practice of spirituality is always present in their way of life, with a strong love of nature and kindness to others.

11. They have a strong faith in their gods to protect them and answer the big questions of life and the hereafter.

12. They use a complimentary medicine approach, combining modern physician and Mind/body interventions.

13. Use prayer and other forms of meditation to reduce elicit the relaxation response and reduce stress.

14. They live a slower, more stress free, natural pace of life characteristic of a non-competitive society.

15. Prioritize supportive social support networks, and the practice helping others which builds a sense of meaning and reduces loneliness.

16. Strong family connection to work together to solve problems and support each other.

17. Strong believers in a holistic approach of mind, body and spirit.

Health Benefits of Okinawan Elders diet and lifestyles.

18. Okinawa death rates per 100,000 people, compared to the US are 82% less for CHD, 27% less for cancer and 35% less from all causes,

19. Okinawa has 34 centenarians per hundred thousand compared to 5 to 10 in US. They have the characteristics associated with healthy aging that are common in other Centenarian studies from other cultures. Above all they have the ability to cope and accept what they can't fix. Other common characteristics include adaptability, Self-confidence, active, independent, relaxed, open and with a desire for social interaction seldom depressed and assertive when necessary.

20. When Okinawans die at average age of 86 for women and 78 for men they are in good Health and death is often classified as old age because no discernible cause can be found. In other words they live longer disability free then Americans.

21. In the US, over 50 percent are overweight and 25 percent are considered obese with the trend skyrocketing. Percentages of overweight are negligible for the elder Okinawans

22. Elderly Okinawa's have amazingly young, clean arteries, low cholesterol [less then 180] and low homocysteine levels [less than 8 plasma total homocysteine mol/l]

23. It is projected by the scientists and authors of 'The Okinawa Program' that the elder Okinawans diet and lifestyles would offer another 5 to 10 years of healthy longevity over the Western diets and lifestyles.

Annual Cancer deaths per 100,000 [1996]

Country	Breast	Prostrate	Colon
Okinawa	6	4	8
Japan	11	8	16
U.S.	33	28	19

Note - According to the major cancer health organizations, no intervention has been found to be as important in overall cancer reduction as cutting back on calories. This includes cancer of the breast, prostate, and colon.

The younger Okinawans

In contrast, the younger Okinawans [below the age of 50] have paid the price of adopting the Western habits of high fat intake and soft living, resulting in the highest level of obesity and highest incidence of cardiovascular diseases in the Japanese Nation. Unfortunately this is a common sad scenario of cultures that have succumbed to westernized environments that prize animal based and processed foods and physical inactivity. Other examples of peoples that have been led on the path of overweight and obesity by their obesity genes, include the Hawaiians, Australian Aborigines and North American natives

In summation

The Elder Okinawan diet and lifestyle health traits are associated with one of the World's leading examples of people with healthy weight and longevity. These traits include a plant based diet with low calorie habits and low body mass index, low animal fat, high soy, fish, moderate alcohol, high physical activity, low stress levels and high family and social networks. The Okinawa Centenarian Study develops strong evidence that the diet and lifestyles of the Okinawa Elders affords protection against most diseases associated with premature aging, including coronary heart disease, cancer and stroke, and gives people their best opportunity at remaining slim and healthy for a longer life. This evidence that it is diet and lifestyles that is more significant than genetics in determining health becomes more obvious when comparing the deteriorated health of the present younger Okinawans that embraced western styles. In addition according to migration studies, when Okinawans are raised abroad or relocate and adopt the habits of their host countries, they also adopt the same diseases and life spans as the people of these host countries.

Rural Chinese Diet

The China Project [Cornell-Oxford-China Diet] conducted in 1983 and 1989-1990 on more than 10,000 families in over 300 villages, was the most massive project on diet and disease ever undertaken. These surveys were undertaken in China because cancer and various other diseases exhibit exceptional geographical localization's and 90% of the people in rural China live their entire lives in the vicinity of their birth and consume diets composed primarily of locally produced food. There are dramatic variances in disease from region to region, cardiovascular disease rates vary by a factor of about 20 fold for one place to another and certain cancer rates may vary by several hundred fold. Across the broad range of villages, the diets of the Chinese people ranged from 6% of their calories in fat to diets that contain significant animal products and up to 24% fat of diets. Comparison data was taken from people on diets that are virtually nil in animal protein to where animal protein is 20 to 30% of the total protein intake. Cholesterol ranged from an average of about 90 to about 170 per 100ml. According the Project directors, such an increase in cholesterol is associated with the emergence of the cancers that increasingly plague the worlds developed nations.

Surprisingly, the study showed that the rural Chinese eat 30% more calories than Americans but that their body mass index is lower and obesity is rare. After adjusting the food intake data to represent a reference male adult involved in the least physical activity and representing the same body weight, total calorie intake of 40 kcal/kg body weigh was about 30% higher in China when compared with an average adult American male however, the body mass index for the Chinese male was about 25% lower [20.5 to 25.8]. More physical activity and a plant-based diet with little fat and animal protein point to the reason as it does in many cultures. It was assumed by study researchers that their bodies are apparently programmed to increase their resting energy use, thereby burning more calories around the clock

Plant Protein is Key to the Cholesterol Dilemma

Abundant studies and trials have shown that blood cholesterol levels can be reduced by replacing dietary animal protein with dietary plant protein. Some the plant protein, particularly soy had impressive ability to reduce blood cholesterol. The dietary patterns in China are strikingly different from Western countries, due to the great variation that could be found in different villages. The same dietary factors which increase blood cholesterol concentrations among Americans also do so in the Chinese, as would be expected. These include increased intakes of dietary fat and animal protein and decreased intakes of dietary fiber and legumes. . The results of the study suggested that the lower the blood cholesterol, the lower the risk for various cancers. Other dietary factors derived from the study indicated that consumption of salt-preserved [pickled] vegetables [a common Chinese food] increase stomach cancer while consumption of fresh vegetables decreases this cancer.

Data from the China study suggest that reducing fat to about 15 % of total calories would prevent 80 to 90 % of chronic degenerative diseases such as cancer, cardiovascular diseases and diabetes before age 65. For example, women who eat diets rich in animal foods reach menarche earlier thereby producing more estrogen over their lifetimes and developing breast cancer a significantly higher rate. According to the study, 'low-fat, high fiber diets are linked with lower levels of female hormones and a lower risk for breast cancer'. Breast cancer, low in China, is greater with consumption of the typical Western diet [high in animal-based foods and fat and low in plant-based foods] which encourages body growth rates to be too rapid and sexual maturation to occur too early.

As the consumption of animal -based foods increases and levels of cholesterol in the blood increase accordingly, the risk for different cancers go up as well, including colon cancer. "In the final analysis, we have strong evidence from this and other studies that nutrition becomes the controlling factor in the development of chronic degenerative diseases "conclude T. Colin Campbell, Director of the Cornell-China-Oxford Project. Campbell goes on to say "Even small intakes of animal foods, which simultaneously alter the intake of countless nutrients and other constituents, is capable of significantly elevating plasma cholesterol and similar biomarkers and thereby elevate the risk of degenerative diseases. Mere tinkering with our diets by consumption of a few low-fat foods or special nutrient supplements, although possible useful under some circumstances, will likely only have minimally useful effects and almost certainly will not be a panacea for disease prevention" He further stressed Americans need to shift to a more plant-based diet.

Health Benefits
Diet and cardiovascular disease

China Project Investigators collected and analyzed body fluids, food samples and mortality data for over 50 diseases, including 7 different cancers, from 65 counties and 130 villages in rural mainland China The combined coronary artery disease mortality rates where inversely associated with the frequency of intake of green vegetables and the findings suggest that even small intakes of foods of animal origin are associated with significant increases in plasma cholesterol concentrations, which in turn are associated with significant increases in chronic degenerative disease mortality rates.

Survey on 65 counties and 130 villages on plant based diets in rural mainland China compared to US

Description	Rural China	U.S.
Fat intake	15% of calories	38 % of calories
Fiber intake	33.3 g/d.	11 g/d
Animal protein intake	10% of U.S.	
Mean serum cholesterol	127 mg/dL	203 mg/dL
Coronary artery disease mortality	6% of U.S.	
Body Mass Index [BMI]	20.5	25.8
Life Expectancy	81.2	76.8
Centenarians per 100,000	34	7

Cornell and Harvard University researchers have teamed up with other experts to unveil an official Asian Diet Pyramid which uses the data collected from the China Project. It reflects the traditional, plan-based rural diets of Asia which research show to be linked to much lower rates of certain cancers, heart disease, obesity, osteoporosis and other chronic, degenerative diseases then those found in the US. The Asian Diet Pyramid emphasizes a wide base of rice, rice products, noodles, breads and grains, preferably whole grain and minimally processed foods. This level is topped by another large band of fruits, vegetables, legumes, nuts and seeds. And then a small amount of vegetable oil and a moderate consumption of plant-based beverages, including tea [preferable black and green] sake, beer and wine also are recommended daily. Small daily serving of dairy products [low fat] or fish are optional, sweets, eggs and poultry are recommended no more than weekly and red meat no more than monthly. Like all diets, to be successful it must be accompanied by daily physical activity.

The nutrient composition of the traditional rural Asian diet is very similar to traditional Mediterranean diets in that both are largely plant-based and animal based foods are consumed on minimum basis of no more than once a month or more often in very small amounts. The main difference is that the Mediterranean diet is higher in total fat, mainly from olive oil. Dairy products, which are largely absent in the diets of Asia, are well regarded in the US for their calcium and are thought by many to inhibit the development of osteoporosis. However, the plant-based, dairy-free diets of much of Asia are linked to a low rate of osteoporosis. In fact Western countries, where calcium is largely taken in the form of dairy products, have significantly higher rates of osteoporosis.

Genetic Influence

In order to determine any genetic influence, a study was performed on the diet and health situation between the Chinese living in North American [US and Canada] and in China. It was noted that the Chinese in North America [NA] have higher rates of many chronic diseases than do Chinese in Asia. Studies on 2488 healthy Chinese residing in NA and China show that the Chinese men in China consumed more calories than those in NA. 2904 versus 2201, with females 2317 versus 1795. The men in China consumed more carbohydrates but less fat. The percent calories from fat were 35% in NA and 22% in China. In contrast the carbohydrates were 62-68% in China and 48% in NA. Chinese in China reported spending more time in vigorous activity, sleeping and walking but less in sitting than in NA. Chinese in China weighed less and were leaner than then the Chinese in NA. The conclusion of the study was that the differences is nutrient intakes, physical activity and body size of Chinese living on two different continents suggest possible explanations for observed higher levels in chronic disease rates in the Chinese NA population.

Conclusion

The protective effect of the nutrients commonly supplied by foods of plant origin was indicated with multiple intake biomarkers disease associations. The indication was that there appears to be no threshold of plant food enrichment or minimization of fat intake beyond which further disease prevention does not occur. These findings suggest that even small intakes of foods of animal origin are associated with significant increases in plasma cholesterol concentrations of which in turn are associated with significant increases in chronic degenerative disease mortality rates. The data from the China Project suggest that the majority of all cancers, cardiovascular diseases and other forms of degenerative illness can be prevented, at least until very old age simply by adopting a plant-based diet.

The Mediterranean Diet

In the early 50ies the American researcher Ancel Keys went to the southern Italian shores to study the notion that heart disease was almost nonexistent in this area, at a time when Americans were experiencing unusually high rates of heart disease. At that time Heart disease was almost unheard of in southern Italy, and then only appeared to occur in a small upper class subculture. This was at a time in the in the 50ies when Americans believed large steak dinners, baked potatoes smothered in butter and a glass of whole milk make a nutritious dinner. Keys was one of the early scientists that demonstrated that diet affected blood cholesterol and blood cholesterol was an indicator of heart disease. . This work led him to spearhead one of the greatest and most influential epidemiological studies of our time, the 'Seven Countries Study.'

The Seven Countries Study examined 13,000 men aged 40 to 59 over a 5 year period in Greece, Italy, Croatia and Serbia, [formerly Yugoslavia] Japan, Finland, the Netherlands and the US. Dietitians stationed in the homes of study subjects took samples of the food for chemical analysis. And after that, an additional 10 year follow up period on more than 10,000 men, examining a range of lifestyle factors in addition. The results provided evidence that the percentage of calories of saturated fat was linked to increased blood cholesterol levels, resulting in an increased risk of coronary heart disease. Those countries with the highest level of saturated fat, namely the US and Finland had the highest rates of heart disease. The US men, Finish and Dutch had heart disease rates that were twice that of Italian men and 4 times that of the Greek and Japanese. In addition the study determined that the rates of all causes of death in the Mediterranean regions where among the lowest in the world.

The first clinical-trial evidence in support of the health benefits of the Mediterranean diet came from the Lyon Diet Heart Study in which 605 patients who had had a myocardial infarction were randomly assigned to a "Mediterranean-style" diet or a control diet resembling the American Heart Association Step 1 diet. Patients in the Mediterranean-style diet group were encouraged to consume more fruits, vegetables and fish, to eat less red meat, and to replace butter and cream with margarine rich in linolenic acid [to mimic the n-3 content of the traditional Cretan diet]. After a mean follow-up of 27 months, the rate of coronary events was reduced by 73 percent and total mortality was reduced by 70 percent in the intervention group.

The term "Mediterranean diet" is somewhat of a misnomer. The countries around the Mediterranean basin all have somewhat different diets, as well as religions and cultures, but all are considerably different from the Western Diet. Their diets differ slightly in the amount of total fat, olive oil, type and amount of meat, wine, fish, milk, cheese. milk, fruits and vegetables. The rates of coronary heart disease and cancer are lower than Western countries, with the lower death rates and longer life expectancy occurring in Greece. On the island of Crete in the 50s and 60s, Greek men enjoyed the longest life expectancy in the world, and men living in other parts of Greece and southern Italy were least likely to develop coronary heart disease. The premature death rate from heart attack for Greek men was 90% lower than that of American men, at that time. This is no true in modern times as their diets, have become increasingly Westernized. More than other Mediterranean diets, the Cretan diet was rich in legumes, fruit and healthy fats that were mostly olive oil. The Cretan diet contained much less meat, but supplied moderate amounts of fish and alcohol, mostly in the form of red wine. The total red meat, poultry and fish consumed on a personal basis in southern Italy was 434 grams [15.5 ounces] per week and in Crete it was about 371 grams [13 ounces] per week. Fish consumption in the Mediterranean region in 1960 varied from 126 grams per person per week in Crete to 519 grams in Spain and 1,057 grams [38 ounces] in Portugal. In Japan which now enjoys the highest life expectancy in the world, fish per-capita consumption has ranged from 532 to 672 grams [19 to 24 ounces] per week over the last 25 years.

The Seven Countries Study reported that men in rural Crete in 1960 were apparently safely consuming 40 % of their energy [calories] in the form of fat - 29% in monounsaturated fat, 8 % in saturated fat and 3 % in polyunsaturated fat. Throughout the Mediterranean, bread was and remains fundamental to the diet. It was hardy, made from natural foods, and enjoyed without butter or margarine. A number of studies of populations in Mediterranean countries where diets consisted largely of foods of plant origin showed low rates of many chronic disease and long life expectancies. Many case control and prospective studies provided further evidence that high consumption of plant foods confers numerous health benefits such as lower rates of, coronary heart disease, several cancers and a number of other diseases. Turning up their noses at plant based foods; Americans in the 1950ies were celebrating their prosperity by eating high fat foods and lying around while people in the Mediterranean area lived with what was available from the land, and what they could afford. Ironically, it was soon to be discovered that the Americans were eating their way to poor health, obesity and degenerative diseases while the Mediterranean's were doing just the opposite

Traditional Mediterranean Diet

Food	Servings	Frequency
Whole grains [breads, pasta, cereals]	8 or more	Daily
Vegetables	3 or more	Daily
Fruit	2 or more	Daily
Legumes [beans, peas]	2 or more	Daily
Dairy [low or nonfat skim milk, yogurt, cheese]	2 or more	Daily
Nuts and seeds	1 oz. or more [1/3 cup]	Daily
Fish [fatty]	6-8 oz. total	Weekly
Lean Animal meats/eggs/poultry	2 or less	Weekly-optional
Olive oil [extra virgin]	2 tablespoon	Daily [15-20% of calories]
Sweets	optional	rarely

A recent major study at 172 centers in Italy finds that eating foods that define the traditional Mediterranean diet leads to cutting the death rate of people who had had a heart attack in half. More than 11.000 people who had had a heart attack were followed for over 6 years after they increased their consumption of fish, fruits, raw and cooked vegetables, and olive oil. Even though there already was regular consumption of these traditional foods, they increased their intake. The study, published in the April 2003 European Journal of Clinical Nutrition, found that there was a linear decrease in mortality with this diet improvement. People who showed the most benefit ate fish as least twice weekly, fruits and vegetables daily and used olive oil regularly. Eating the combination of foods, rather than one food, appeared to provide the most benefits.

Evidence that Mediterranean-style diet containing olive oil is beneficial to health

1. A diet rich in complex carbohydrates and fiber and whose fat source is primarily monounsaturated fatty acids as found in the olive oil rich Mediterranean-styles diet lowers LDL cholesterol and is associated with a low incidence of CHD

2. Epidemiological studies provide evidence that in countries where a Mediterranean style diet is consumed, colon cancer incidence is low compared with Northern European countries

3. The traditional Mediterranean style diet has been shown to predispose to a lower blood pressure compared with typical "Western diets.

4. Epidemiological data show a strong inverse relationship between carbohydrates intake and relative body weight. Due to its high content of complex carbohydrates the Mediterranean diet lower energy content than a high fat diet making it more suitable for prevention of obesity.

5. The beneficial health effect of olive oil is due to both its high content of monounsaturated fatty acids and its high content of antioxidative substances. When substituted for saturated fatty acids it reduces total LDL cholesterol without reducing the levels of HDL cholesterol.

6. The Lyon Diet Heart Study in patients recovering from heart attack showed a Mediterranean diet high in monounsaturated fatty acids, such as in olive oil, protects against CHD

7. A study published in *Circulation: The Journal of the American Heart Association* described a four year study in France following more than 600 men and women who had had one

heart attack. They found those consuming the traditional Mediterranean diet had a 50 to 70% lower risk of a second heart attack than those in a control group. The control group consumed a typical Western diet, where almost 34% of calories came from fat and almost 12% from saturated fat. The Mediterranean diet averaged 30% from fat and only 8% from saturated fat.

Regrettably, the traditional Mediterranean Diet is going the way of other developing countries as they join the pandemic of over-weight and obesity. Dietary patterns in Greece and other Mediterranean countries are changing rapidly, with increased consumption of saturated fat and refined carbohydrates. This coupled with reduced physical activity, follows the obesity gene equation and this former HALL country joins the march to unhealthy weight and poorer health.

Comparison of diets, lifestyles and health of the traditional HALL peoples and the US today

DIET	U.S. currently	Okinawa Elders [1] About 1970	Rural Chinese Traditional [2] About 1980	Mediterranean Traditional [3] About 1960
Fat - % of diet	40	24	14.5	20-40% (4)
Saturated fat - %diet		7		7-8
Animal Protein - % of diet		15	10% of U.S.	
Carbohydrates	48	61		
Fiber - grams/day	11		33	
Processed foods	Frequent	Rare	Rare	Rare
HEALTH				
Healthy Life Expectancy HALE 2001 [6]	67.6	73.6		70.4

BMI	25.8	20	20.5	
Calories versus US	100%	80%	130%	
Cholesterol	203 avg.	Under 180	127	
Heart Disease death rates	100	18	40	55 (5)
Stroke death rates	28	35	40	60 (5)
Cancer death rates	132	97	126	125 (5)
All causes death rates	520	335	393	455 (5)
Overweight	50%	Negligible	Negligible	Negligible
Obesity	25%	Negligible	Negligible	Negligible
LIFESTYLES				
Physical activity	Low	high	High	high
Stress compared to US		lower	Lower	Lower
Family comp to US		more	more	more

Sources and notes

1. Okinawa Elders - The Okinawa Program is a 25 year centenarian study-later 20th century
2. Rural China source - The Cornell-Oxford-China Diet, et, al in 1983-1990
3. Mediterranean source - The Seven Countries Study, et al about 1960
4. Mostly Olive Oil
5. Per 100,000 per WHO 1996
6. HALE - Healthy Life Expectancy- WHO World Report 2001 -HALE is based on life expectancy, but includes an adjustment for time spent in poor health.

In the last few decades, the traditional HALL peoples have become more westernized in their diets and lifestyles and joined the overweight and obesity pandemic. Their comparative disease protection, as expected, is diminishing, however, for the time being they still live longer and are disabled less than Americans.

Age-standardized death rates per 100,000 [1997]

	All Cancer	Breast Cancer	Prostate Cancer	Circulatory diseases	Heart Disease	Cerebro -vascular	All Causes
US							
Males	176		19	271	144	37	722
Females	121	21		172	78	32	463
JAPAN [1]							
Males	179		7	159	42	72	556
Females	87	7		96	21	46	295
GREECE							
Males	167		12	277	99	83	632
Females	89	17		210	42	83	414
SINGA-PORE							
Males	184		7	241	142	65	670
Females	19	17		177	93	57	443
ITALY [1995]							
Males	199		14	248	93	62	673
Females	105	22		162	44	50	388

[1] Death rates for the Elder Japanese in the Okinawa Study, was about 15 to 20% less for each disease then Japan.

Source - World Health Organization and the Okinawa Program 25 year study.

CHAPTER FIVE

The obesity genes
eating [Ogd] program

1. The bottom line
2. Avoid these foods
3. The skinny on fats
4. Food choices at a glance
5. Serving sizes
6. Recommended food groups
7. Preparing vegetables
8. Helpful hints
9. Eat multiple meals
10. Summary

1. The bottom line

The OBESITY GENES eating plan is designed for eating enjoyment, and not a test of will power. .After you have sufficiently practiced the epigenetic interventions in Chapter 6, you will prefer to eat these recommended foods. Here you will find enticing vegetable and grain-based dishes from the Healthiest and Longest Lived [HALL] people. These delightful dishes can and will play a growing role in your meals while food derived from animals will play a decreasing role. Vegetables, fruits, and whole grains contain vitamins, minerals and phytochemicals that help fight free radicals, those unstable oxygen molecules that drill holes in our body's cellular walls damaging the DNA genetic material within. Free radical damage sets us up for debilitating, disabling diseases. The basic premise of the free radical theory is that the combustion of oxygen in our cells that keeps us alive and active also spins off by products called oxygen free radicals, which also attack good cells, until the cells become dysfunctional. . The cellular damage accumulates over the years until enough cell are destroyed to the point of fatal diseases. The perpetual but futile struggle of individual cells to stay alive and function normally in the face of chemical disintegration is the genesis of aging and all its consequences. While controversial, some experts' estimate 80 to 90 % of all degenerative disease involves free radical activity. The body's defense against free radicals includes anti-oxidants, which neutralize these oxygen radicals, rendering them harmless. A number of studies suggest that anti-oxidants affect the progress of some diseases more common in middle and old age, including atherosclerosis, cancer, cataracts, Alzheimer's disease, and Parkinson's disease. In theory, the probability of developing free radical diseases, including aging, should be decreased by reducing metabolic rate and oxidation. [calorie restriction and antioxidants]. And indeed, this is the case for calorie restriction, where it has been repeatedly demonstrated in animals that food restriction remarkably reduces aging.

The health of the HALL peoples gives credibility to the supposition that natural antioxidants from foods such as antioxidant rich vegetables and fruits especially work to protect us from premature aging, cancer, hardening of the arteries and other degenerative diseases. The phytochemicals within these healthy foods contain names like beta-carotene, lycopene, and sulforaphane, substances that strengthen the body's immune system, reducing free radicals and protecting us from carcinogens. It's important to eat a wide variety of plant foods because scientific research indicates that these plant substances seem to be synergistic. The typical and traditional American diet contains a large piece of meat and a small serving of vegetables and some form **of** carbohydrate, typically in the form of potatoes or rice. This combination of food usually contains too many calories and provides too few healthy nutrients to prevent chronic illness or help people maintain healthy weight.

On the other hand, the OGD is built around tasty [if not now, it soon will be after mental conditioning takes effect] vegetables, grains, and fruit. It more than provides the five to ten servings of vegetables and fruits that the HALL peoples typically consume. On the MMD diet you can fill up on fruits and vegetables, but you do have to change the proportion of the types of foods that are on your plate. You have to substantially decrease the amount of animal-based foods and increase the amount of plant-based foods. A healthy proportion to aim for initially is about two-thirds or more of vegetables, fruits, whole grains, and beans and less than one third from animal based products. As your food preferences are retrained by EMP Behavioral program, animal based food will become less desirable and more occasional...

Calorie counting or hunger pangs are not required by the MMD diet, because plant foods tend to be rich in nutrients and relatively low in calories. You can eat all you want from the vegetable list and as many as ten servings a day from the grain list. Because these foods contain a lot of fiber, they tend to fill you up, thereby reducing calories without inducing hunger pains. Initially, the diet does ask you to limit your servings of low-fat, calcium-rich dairy foods such as yogurt, cheese and sour cream to two or three servings a day, and to limit your servings of chicken, meat, poultry and eggs to less than one serving a day. Sweets from refined carbohydrates to be limited to 0 to 3 servings per week...

2. Avoid these foods

The OGD plan is aimed at avoiding certain foods. As is no surprise, they are those simple carbohydrates typically using unbleached and enriched grains and refined sugar, along with saturated fats, trans-fats and a number of questionable chemicals. Examples of such foods include: cake, cookies, croissants, doughnuts, pastries, pie crusts and other typical bakery products. Packaged snacks such as potato chips, tortilla chips, and corn chips, and any processed food that contains white flour, sugar, saturated fats, oils and trans-fats] are also to be avoided. Generally speaking, any food that is processed is 'guilty until proven innocent'. Recently, there has been an attempt by the food industry to reduce animal fats and increase whole grain content, while still providing traditional Western tastes. Although this is still a work in progress, some packaged snacks show promise.

3. The Skinny on Fats

Although the OGD program is a low fat diet, it is not to say that fats aren't vital for life, in fact the majority of every cell in our body and the brain is fat. This is what makes it is critical to know what kind of fats are healthy. Saturated fats generally come from animal products and have been shown to increase cholesterol, and are linked to heart disease. Whereas, monounsaturated fats [i.e. olive and canola oil] are healthy, as demonstrated by the HALL peoples and extensive studies.

Guidelines for fats and oils

    a. Reduce consumption of saturated fats
    b. Omit partially hydrogenated fats as much as possible
    c. Minimize polyunsaturated oils, especially when cooking
    d. Use unrefined monounsaturated oils
    e. Store oil in glass containers in the dark, preferably refrigerated
    f. Choose cold-pressed olive oil over other extractive methods.

Essential fatty acids are Omega 3 and 6 fatty acids. Omega 3 goes rancid rapidly and food processing removes most of it. Omega

3 fatty acid decreases platelet aggregation suppresses inflammation and helps keeps blood vessels clear, greatly reducing the risk of cardiovascular diseases. Omega 6 does just the opposite and increases platelet aggregation, stimulates inflammation, but in the right ratios they balance each other. Good sources of Omega 3 are fatty fish, and flax seed oil, Good sources of Omega 6 are vegetables oils, such as corn oil and safflower oil. . Historically diets were balanced the balance was in the order of 1 to 1 to 1 to 4 in Omega 3 to Omega 6. Current average diets are now unbalanced with an estimated at 1 to 30 ratio between Omega 3 and Omega 6. This tremendous change over the decades from traditional diets is inconsistent with HALL diets and modern nutritional science. Hence the emphasis to add Omega 3 to modern diets.

The traditional diets, consumed by peoples with the lowest incidence of heart disease, are certain Mediterranean and Asian countries... The Mediterranean area diet is not typically referred to as low fat, and in fact the highest fat consumers are on the Island of Crete where their diet is 40% fat, [mostly in olive oil] and they have traditionally enjoyed one of the lowest incidences of heart disease in the world. On the other extreme, the mainland Japanese diet is one of the lowest in fat, about 10% and they have one of the longest healthy life span in the world, despite their high level of stress due to high density population, extreme level of industrial pollution, and high rates of cigarette smoking. The elder Okinawans' eat a similar diet, as the Japanese, but they are relative free from stress living, and they enjoy the highest concentration of centenarians. While the Japanese diet is significantly different from the American diet, the traditional Mediterranean is not so far afield. It is low in meat, which is eaten occasionally, high in fish and vegetables, and includes some dairy products; in the form of yogurt and fresh cheeses. Whole grain bread is a mainstay and significant amounts of their dietary fat are from olive oil. Their diet is has been frequently studied and several decades ago was correlated with a low incidence of heart disease and cancer. However, in the later part of the 20th century it has become more westernized, and their healthy resistance to major diseases has trended downward.

4. OGD Food choices at a glance

Food	Servings [1]	Frequency
Mostly whole grains [breads, pasta, cereals, brown rice, noodles]	7 or more	Daily
Vegetables	7 or more	Daily
Fruit	2 or more	Daily
Legumes [beans, peas]	2 or more	Daily
Dairy [low or nonfat skim milk, yogurt, cheese]	1-2	Daily
Animal meats/eggs/poultry	0-2	Weekly-optional
Fish – Salmon, trout, sardines	6-8 oz. total	Weekly
Other Omega-3 [flaxseed, soy products]	1	Daily
Nuts and seeds	1 oz. [1/3 c cup]	Daily
Olive oil [extra virgin]	1-2 tbl	Daily
Tea [green, black, oolong]		
Wine, beer, sake	Optional	1-2 drinks/day
Sweets	optional	rarely

Notes;

[1]. While the serving sizes are small, for those who only require a low level of calories it is not necessary to eat all the serving indicated.

[2] Eat a variety of vegetables and fruits.

[3] About 55% to 65% of diet to be carbohydrates [the great majority to be complex -minimize simple carbohydrate intake such as sugar.

[4] Eat about 20 to 30 % of diet calories from fats [the majority from olive and canola oil -keep saturated and trans-fats to less than 5% of total calories].

[5] About 10 to 15% of diet calories to high quality protein, such as beans [minimal animal fat]

SERVING SIZES
VEGETABLES
1 cup of raw leafy vegetables   1/2 cup of other vegetables cooked or chopped raw   1/4 cup of vegetable juice
WHOLE GRAINS
1/2 cup of cooked cereal, rice, or pasta   1 oz. of ready to eat cereal 1 slice of bread or 1/2 bagel
FRUITS
1/2 cup of chopped, cooked or canned fruit   1 medium apple, banana orange, pear, or plum   1/4 cup of fruit juice
DAIRY
1-1/2 oz. of low fat cheese   1 cup of low fat or skim milk   1 cup of low fat or fat free yogurt
ADDITIONAL OMEGA 3- FOODS
1 tablespoon of ground flaxseed   2 tablespoons of chopped walnuts   2 tablespoons of soy nuts
1 teaspoon of canola oil   1 cup cereal with flaxseed [Uncle Sam]
MEAT/POULTRY/EGGS
2-3 oz. of cooked poultry   2-3 oz. of cooked lean meat 1 egg

Nutrient Conversions

1 gram = 1,000 mg = 1,000,000 micrograms
5 grams - 1 teaspoon
14 grams - 1/2 ounce - 1 tablespoon = 3 teaspoons
28 grams - 1 ounce - 2 tablespoons

7. Preparing vegetables

As a general rule it is wise to plan ahead and buy only as many vegetables as your family can eat within three or four day or else you will end up with limp broccoli, mushy mushrooms, and wilted fruit. To guarantee getting the best nutrition, eat many vegetables raw or cook them as close as you can to serving time. Prolonged exposure to air and sunlight can diminish their nutritional value. For best buys and fresher fruit and vegetables, try visiting a local farmers market or save money and plant your own vegetable garden if you have a home with a backyard.

Don't overcook vegetables. There are many cooking methods for vegetables.

- Steaming preserves more nutrients and their flavor and texture more than any other conventional technique. For proper steaming, place vegetables in a steamer basket above boiling water. Tightly cover the pan to keep in the steam. Cook until vegetables are tender crisp. Another good cooking technique is blanching which involves plunging the vegetables in boiling water for one to three minutes then quickly transferring them to ice water to stop the cooking process. Unlike boiling, this method preserves the color and texture of vegetables. Blanching is an especially good cooking method for hard vegetables such as carrots, broccoli, cauliflower, asparagus, and peppers.
- Braising is a method where one slowly cooks vegetables with only a small amount of liquid which is then used a sauce for the vegetables. The braising liquid can be broth or water enhanced with chopped tomatoes, onions, garlic or herbs for flavor.
- Stir-frying is a popular, quick method of cooking vegetables. The heat is kept relatively high and cut vegetables are turned continuously over the heat until they are crisp tender. It's best to cut the vegetable in relatively small pieces to ensure that they are all cooked to proper texture. Use a wok or a heavy skillet and don't put the vegetables in until the pan is hot or the food will absorb too much cooking oil and stick. Remember to use olive or canola oil...
- Roasting is a good method for cooking potatoes, sweet potatoes, eggplant, peppers, winter squash, carrots, and tomatoes. The dry heat preserves the flavor of vegetables better than steaming. Roast vegetables in a shallow baking pan at 400 to 450 degrees until tender.

- Grilling brings out a slightly smoky flavor in certain vegetables such as sweet peppers, tomatoes, large mushrooms, potatoes, and corn. Brush or spray those veggies with a little oil to prevent drying or marinate them in a low fat dressing prior to grilling.
- Frozen vegetables can be quickly defrosted and cooked in microwave ovens. Rotate the vegetables during cooking to prevent drying and uneven hot spots.

8. **Helpful hints**

- When cooking with olive or canola oil, or using them on food, spray on instead of pouring.
- Drinking water before meals will reduce appetite
- Eat chunky rather than finely chopped salads and pureed soups to feel fuller.
- Read labels to be aware of the calories and trans-fats in your choices.
- Leave the table a little hungry, by reducing portion sizes, or avoiding the clean plate syndrome. If the hunger won't go away later, you can fill up on the after meal snacks of fruits and raw vegetables.
- Eat slowly to allow your satiety sensors to operate before you have overeaten.
- Eat foods high in unrefined carbohydrates and fiber to help keep calories low without a feeling of starvation. A sort of a 'eat more weigh less' strategy.
- When overcooking the amounts recommended, use for another meal.
- When eating at a restaurant, plan to take out a doggie bag, since the portion served will usually be a diet buster of unhealthy proportions.
- Drink tea at least once a day. Both green and black tea has been shown to reduce the risk of several types of cancers. Choose low fat food. Fat has a low satiety value, which means

that you have to eat more to feel full or satisfied. It also stimulates your fat instinct so the chances of overeating will increase.

- Choose foods high in fiber. The more fiber, the more filling it will be on the fewest number of calories. Plant foods meet these criteria. Fibrous foods also slow absorption of sugars to maintain fat burning at high levels to contribute to weight loss.

- Choose foods with least amount of simple sugars. Foods with high sugar cause your body to reduce its fat burning in order to burn the excess sugar in your blood thereby retaining the fat in your tissues. Simple sugars are most common in processed foods and most foods made from white flour, such as white bread and bakery goods.

- Don't over eat nuts. While nuts are a healthy food, in that they contain good fats that are heart healthy, are relatively high in protein, have cholesterol-lowering phytochemicals and fiber, they are high in calories. A single ounce, not more than a couple of tablespoons has 160 to 180 calories depending on the variety. Consequently, this must be considered on a weight loss program.

- Put a reminder on the fridge door - do you really want and need to eat what you are thinking about.

- Buy only in the smallest quantities. The less there is to eat, the less you will eat. More trips to the grocery store will present fewer opportunities to eat.

- Reduce the portions on your plate. Numerous studies have shown that most people tend to eat whatever in on their plate.

- Reduce opportunities to eat

9. Eat multiple meals

Eating several times a day accomplishes two fundamental goals, first you aren't hungry all the time which means that your fat desire slumbers. Second, you keep your insulin levels low which keeps you burning fat all day long, Our ancestors basically grazed, eating as many as twelve or more serving of vegetables and fruits per day. While the average American eats only two meals a day which promotes weight retention and weight gain. A substantial number of studies have indicated that grazing - eating 6 to 8 small meals a day is better than eating the same number of calories in three or less, large meals. By reducing the levels of insulin in the blood and other health benefits. Starving you and then gorging on a large meal causes substantial stress on the digestive system, including high levels of insulin in the blood, with can lead to diabetes as well as other health problems.

CHAPTER SIX

While the preceding tips and information will precondition you and point you in direction of healthy weight loss, without modifying your obesity genes you will soon be back to where you started, but not for long. The only way to long term weight control is to change the obesity genes that are the major cause of the problem. And this can only be done with epigenetic modifiers

HOW THE EPIGENETIC
MODIFIER PROGRAM MAKES IT WORK.

1. The goals of the program
2. The biology of the Program
3. ...The EMP 6 month outli
4. The first month plan-4 acts
5. What is mindfulness?
6. Following your breath
7. Act 1-Mindful eating
8. Act 2-Eat from OGD food group
9. .Act 3 -Consume less calories
10. Act 4-Burn 100 calories a day –
11. Activity calories table
12. Daily Acts Journal
13. Month two –Changing eating habits
14. Understanding EMP Self Hypnosis

    a. What is self-hypnosis?
    b. Your conscious and subconscious mind
    c. Changing eating habits and reasons for eating
    d. Install posthypnotic eating suggestions
    e. Components of the EMP plan

15. Self-Hypnosis induction script

The primary goal is to adopt the basic eating habits and physical activity of the traditional HALL peoples, in a practical and cost effective way. This genetic modification requires a change in subconscious eating by becoming more conscious in order to change your beliefs and perceptions. This process will take a committed effort, of living in the present, where you are free from being controlled by your unconscious mind and its genetic programs. As you become slimmer and experience more energy to do the things you want, you will enjoy life more; have better health and more freedom from chronic stress and pain.

1. The goals of the program

    a. **Change learned food preferences** to adopt the food preferences of the HALL peoples. While we won't eat what we don't enjoy very long, fortunately our food preferences are mostly learned habits. And learned habits can be changed by epigenetic programs to modify behavior. The Epigenetic Modifier program mental conditioning through knowledge, mindfulness, self-hypnotherapy and other epigenetic modifiers

    b. **Satisfy your genetic desire for fats and sweets** – Acknowledge and accept the programming of our 'Obesity Genes" for fats, sweets, and quantity and substitute healthy fats, and natural sweets.

    c. **Satisfy your genetic drive for more calories** – Satisfy the hunger of your 'Obesity Genes' for more calories by mindfully eating unlimited amounts of low calorie healthy foods, such as fruits and vegetables, which you will soon prefer.

d. Become aware of your subconscious eating programs – become aware of other reasons for eating, such as opportunistic, social, emotional, etc. and once they are made conscious they can be prevented by being in the state of mindfulness, [frequently referred to as living in the moment]. Understandably, in order to make any change, you must first be aware of what you are doing.

e. Overcome our genetic drive for lower activity levels – change our subconscious programs for physical inactivity by self-hypnosis and imagery in order to find enjoyable ways to increase physical activity.

f. Changing your eating behavior in a practical way. No matter how effective the program, the fact is that most people have a limited amount of time and opportunities to invest in a self-improvement program. To insure that the epigenetic modifier program is practical as well as effective, it is designed so that no more than 5 to 15 minutes a day is required, exclusive of exercise.

2. The biology of the Epigenetic Modifier Program

The effectiveness of the EMP depends on being able to change your eating habits in a convenient and practical way. This ability evolves from the power of your conscious mind to modify your genes thus changing your biology. Until recently the process by which the mind can change your biology has been unclear, until recent research on epigenetic mechanisms. It is well known that the placebo effect is a classic example of how the mind can influence the biology of the body. However until recently, the chemical and genetic mechanisms were not known. But now the rapidly expanding science of epigenetics, is resulting in forms of 'Genetic Engineering'

Until recent research in genetics, most scientists thought that the human body was a "biochemical machine 'programmed' by its genes, and that our abilities, such as artistic and intellectual, and our health, such as diseases, depressions, etc. were genetically programmed. But now, stimulated by the Human Genome Project a radically new understanding has emerged. It is now recognized that the environment, and more specifically, our perception (interpretation) of the environment, directly controls the expression of our genes, through a process known as epigenetic control. This new perspective of human biology incorporates the role of a mind and spirit in all healing, for when we change our perception or beliefs we send totally different messages to our cells and reprogram their expression. This may explain why some people seem to have had spontaneous remissions or recover from disabilities thought to be permanent. It is thought that when the mind perceives that the environment is safe, the cells are focused on the growth and maintenance of the body. However, under stressful situations, the cells change their focus and energy resources to adopt a protective mode and cells used to sustain growth are diverted to systems that provide protection during periods of stress. .

The principle source of stress is the system's 'central voice,' the unconscious mind, but there are two separate minds that create the 'central voice.' The conscious mind is a creative, problem solving, decision making mind and only operates in the present. The subconscious mind is like a recorder of our genetic programs, instincts and life experiences. The subconscious mind is verbalized by the 'voice in our head' and controls our behavior when we are not in our conscious mind, which is most of the time.

Popular diet programs attempt to sell the concept that by using will power, we can override negative eating habits. But this is not the case, as hopeful dieters have found out. If you could use will power, you would need to keep a constant vigil on your eating habits, because the moment you lapse in consciousness, the subconscious mind will automatically play its old eating habit program. The subconscious mind can be thought of as a recorder that plays back genetic drives and epigenetic life experiences. Consequently there is no discernment whether the subconscious behavioral program is good or bad.

The subconscious mind has much greater power then the conscious mind, as an information processor. Neuroscientists state that the conscious mind only provides about 5%, while the sub-conscious provides about 95% of our daily cognitive activity during the day. So, no matter how determined you are your will be unable to change the eating habits programed in your subconscious, Will-power against genes – no contest. Since you can't change the eating habits locked in your unconscious mind, you need to create eating habits in your conscious mind, which are not controlled by your obesity genes. To become more conscious, the EMP Program uses mindful eating practices and other conscious acts as shown in Phase 1 of the program. Secondly, we use proven self-hypnosis and imaging program that has been shown effective in reprogramming habits. Our programs are specifically designed to reduce obesity gene influence and change eating habits.

3. The Epigenetic Modifier Plan - 6 month outline

Month one - perform and journal 4 daily acts –
Act 1 - Mindful eating. Eat one daily meal mindfully. This act focuses on the practice of mindfulness. The purpose is to take our mind's attention away from our random scattered thoughts so that we can become aware of our eating patterns and eat Consciously.
Act 2 -Eat one OGD meal daily. Educates on the fundamental food types and eating guidelines
Act 3 - Calorie reduction - Practice consuming 5-10% less calories at one meal. Lists suggestions for calorie reduction
Act 4 - Additional physical activity - Burn an extra 100 calories daily. Describes various activities and their associated calories.

Month - Two – Changing eating habits

1. Read the EMP self-hypnosis plan daily until understood
2. Practice Verbal suggestions daily
3. Practice self-hypnosis procedure-at least weekly from script
4. Act 1- Eat one mindful meal daily
5. Act 2 – Eat one meal using OGD food groups -daily

6. Eat 5-10% less calories at largest meal
7. Burn an extra 200 calories

Month – Three – Reinforcing eating habits

1. Practice using post hypnotic suggestions for healthy eating patterns
2. Practice affirmations to develop healthy subconscious programs.
3. Practice self-hypnosis procedure at least twice weekly
4. Eat at least 2 mindful meals daily
5. Eat at least 1 meal from OGD food groups
6. Burn at least 300 calories

Months four and five – Confirming new eating habits

1. Practice self-hypnosis induction at least 3 times a week
2. Practice affirmations daily
3. Practice suggestion triggers 3 times weekly
4. Eat all meals mindfully.
5. Eat all meals from OGD food groups or menus
6. Burn at least 300 extra calories daily or 1,500 weekly

Month six – New lifetime eating and activity habits

1. Practice EMP self-hypnosis induction as necessary
2. Practice mindful eating as a habit for all meals
3. Burn at least 1,500 extra calories weekly
4. Eat all meals from OGD food groups

GRADUATION

The detailed procedures for the above steps follow below. While the 6 month time line is normal, you may have reason to adjust them, depending on your personal circumstances. If you have adhered to this program, your new eating habits should be having their effects on your waist line and quality of life. If this is not the case, return to the step with which you feel comfortable, and move thru the steps of the program again as you are able.

4. First month Plan

Perform and Journal the 4 acts daily for one month

ACT 1 - MINDFUL EATING

Background

The first step in the EMP program is the practice of mindfulness. This will allow you to become aware of your eating, activity habits and patterns relative to the OGD fundamental food and activity guidelines. The state of mindfulness will empower you to reduce unnecessary subconscious eating, and inactivity, such as: opportunistic, social, emotional, and psychological. This epigenetic technique of mental conditioning is widely used and is frequently referred to as 'living in the moment'. The point being that in order to make any change, you must first be aware of what you are doing. The practice of mindfulness is critical throughout the EMP program to make you aware of your environment and thoughts in the present moment, so that you can exert some control of your mind, which obviously is essential in epigenetic programs.

5. What is mindfulness?

From a viewpoint of Eastern consciousness the Western state of consciousness seems like an extended dream rather than then being awake to the fullness of life. The practice of mindfulness is the means by which we can wake up from this dream life and participate in life as it unfolds moment by moment. Mindfulness is not a belief or tradition, religious or scientific, but rather a practical, natural way to be aware of your life, moment by moment. The practice of mindfulness is nothing more than being non-judgmentally aware of your thoughts, feelings and environment in the present moment. If we are not living in the present moment, our thoughts are in the past or the future where we can only experience the worries and fears that our imagination generates. In this dream world, our imaginary fears, anxieties and concerns generate their attached emotions which usually have a negative spin, and we suffer needlessly and become ineffective. The uninitiated think that meditation is a way to run away from your problems, but the opposite is true. Instead it is a way to see your problems more clearly and thereby permit a realistic perspective of them so that you can resolve and accept them.

For instance consider the problems involved in weight management. First we must realize that our attraction to food is complex and stems not only from our obesity genes, but also from subconscious, emotional and psychological desires in addition to its natural purpose of providing a healthy energy source to fuel our body. When we are totally present, we are better able to make conscious logical decisions for healthy eating, rather than letting our subconscious attraction of unhealthy foods dominate us. Similar to eating unhealthy foods, overeating does not stem from a healthy fulfillment of our current biological needs, but rather genetic predisposition's from a historic era, as well as an attempt to satisfy emotional and psychological desires and opportunistic subconscious eating.

To do just about anything effectively, you need to focus your awareness. The most creative and productive people in every field and area have the ability to block out distractions and completely immerse themselves in their task. This state of total awareness and focusing is the state in which world records are set, visionary concepts are developed and where we are at our peak efficiency. It is in this state that we have the best chance at making our most healthy decisions on weight management, as well as healthy longevity. When we can bring all of our energies to bear on whatever task is at hand, whether it is witnessing the beauty of some delight of nature, washing the dishes or doing our taxes, we become the most effective, appreciative, and productive we can be. The EMP program teaches the practice of the power of mindfulness to become aware of your subconscious, emotional and opportunistic eating patterns and once they are made conscious you will have the power to end or modify them

To the American mindset we expect to get something for our efforts, otherwise we think we are wasting our time. In the OGD program the management of a healthy weight is the fruit resulting from the combination of mindfulness and knowledge of the OGD basic eating program. Our goal is to go into a state of mindfulness whenever food is present or involved. When we are consciously aware of what and why we want to eat, we are taking a conscious action for healthy eating. Following are the basic steps of mindfulness to start practice. Remember, anyone can become mindful of their environment, as this is a natural part of part of our genetic design. To focus our mind so that it is restricted from bouncing around with a stream of different thought is the object of the exercise.

Mindfulness saves time and increases efficiency - One of the main reasons we fail to practice mindfulness is that we don't think there is time in our already busy schedules. But the reality is that the practice of mindfulness gives more productive time then it takes. Busy persons, in a hurry to make a living, attend to others; make a meeting or appointment, and so on, doesn't feel they have the time to practice mindfulness. The reality is that when you keep your attention focused on the task at hand, you can handle any situation that arises in a manner much more efficiently, then when you are multitasking or doing it while dreaming of the future or the past. When we are not in control of ourselves we will not be as effective as we can be and our work is of less value. When your mind wanders from the task at hand, this is your cue to return to following your breath. In mindfulness, the power stems from practice.

That doesn't mean that you just have to add one more thing to an already overloaded schedule, but rather that you will be able to do all the tasks better and more efficiently, because you are awake and able to concentrate your energy on your work. Ironically, by being more efficient you will gain time. Another way that mindfulness gives you more time is by conserving your energy. The fatigue that grips many of us at the end of the workday is not a natural tiredness, but the product of a day filled with wasted thoughts and feelings of anxiety and worry, not to speak of anger and resentments openly expressed or inwardly held. These negative mental states probably do more to sap energy than anything else. In contrast, the trained mindful person moves through their tasks aware and alert. The task at hand receives its due share of your energy, but none is wasted in anxiety, fantasy, or smoldering resentment. Even at the end of a full day's work your store of energy is not exhausted

6. Following your breath–Your breath is your link to bring you back to a state of mindfulness. Since your breath is always with you, you can practice mindfulness at your convenience. In the privacy of your home, in a nature setting, waiting in line, almost whatever you happen to be doing. Since mindfulness makes you more alert to what you are doing and thinking, it makes you more effective at just about anything you do. Be ever mindful that the breath is the bridge to your mind, and the most direct link is when all breathing is done with the diaphragm. When first beginning to notice your breath, breathe normally and count the length in and then out, then you will know the length of your breath. Then try to extend the exhalation to more counts then you will empty your lungs of more air.

As previously discussed, to be in the moment is to pay attention and be aware of this moment and everything connected with this moment. This initially is an act of will, and you will soon find your mind drifting somewhere else as you are seeking what seems to be more interesting or productive. Until sufficient practice is undertaken to make mindfulness a habit, this will be a frequent occurrence. The breath is the means to bring back your wandering mind. Being aware of our breathing makes us aware that we are here now. You might say, our breath is the metronome of our life, and it responds to balance changes in bodily states. It sets the rhythm for our body, and is always there. When you are aware that you're consciousness is elsewhere, gently bring it back by centering on your breath. Feel your normal breath coming into your body and leaving your body. Try to be aware of each breath for its full duration, the entire in-breath, and the entire out-breath. Do not try to control your breath-just be aware of it. If your breathing gets shallower, let it be shallow, if it gets faster or slower, let it. The breath regulates itself.

Don't try to force it or change it, but just feel it and be aware of it. Using the breath as an anchor to bring us back can be done in an instant, by just paying attention to it. Following your breath means making your breath calm and even. Initially, to train yourself to follow your breath, and block out the usual stream of mind chatter-you can focus on counting. Counting one on inhaling and two on exhaling, three on inhaling and so forth, continuing up to ten, and starting over again. Another popular technique is to breathe in through your nose to the count of 4, hold your breath for a count of 6 and exhale slowly through your mouth for a count of 8. There are many suitable ways of following your breath and whatever works best for you is the one you should use. Your breath should be light and smooth, so that a person next to you would not hear it. Our breath is the bridge from body to our mind and allows building up of endless vitality.

Our natural ability to be mindful comes from our human design of being able to only think of one thing at a time. When we focus on one thing, other thoughts are blocked out from our consciousness, and for that instant, we are incapable of worry, desiring something else or any other motivation. Since this is a characteristic of our human nature all healthy people have the ability to concentrate and be mindful.

As you try several different techniques of following your breath, you will find one more comfortable than others. For those who have difficulty in choosing, the standard technique taught by the EMP program is as follows. Breathe in the left nostril on the mental count of one and out the right nostril on the count of two. Continue breathing in the left nostril on odd counts and out the right nostril on even counts, until you get to the count of 10 and then start over again. Feel the air passing through each nostril. The rate of breathing is normal and not to be forced. You will be aware that you are focusing on your breath coming in and going out, when your mind is empty of your normal random stream of thoughts.

7. Act 1-Mindful Eating

Start mindfully - Start your day on waking with a half-smile by relaxing your facial muscles and following your breath. Be mindful of each action in your morning routine, while following your breath.

Savor the food −. Eating mindfully is being aware of the texture and taste of each bite, so that you become fully aware of the food you are eating and add to its enjoyment Eat very slowly, breaking down each movement so that you are aware of each mouthful and the nuance and sensational of texture, sound, taste and movement. For instance, if you are eating peas, initially be aware of each pea, its shape, firmness, and flavor. This, of course doesn't have to be for every pea, but just enough to be aware of each type of food. After a few peas, try a spoon full of another food, and be aware of its characteristics.

Eating in this way not only allows you to enjoy your meal better, but it also will result in Consuming fewer calories, since it gives your natural biological systems time to produce a satiety signal before you have over eaten. It also reduces subconscious unnecessary eating, such as opportunistic, emotional and various psychologically motivated eating.

Making mindful eating a habit

Find some way to remind you to become mindful whenever you are thinking of, or are around food. Initially it could be a string around your finger, wearing your ring rotated 90 or 180 degrees, or some other method of keeping it in your mind so that a 'bell' goes off in your head when you are around food. When you are working on the self-hypnosis scripts you will be able to use posthypnotic suggestions to remind you to become mindful, until it becomes a habit.

Mindful eating is the best defense against opportunistic, emotional, social and other forms of subconscious eating. An added benefit is that the practice of mindfulness will also reduce worry and anxiety, by 'living in the moment'. Mindfulness should be practiced several times a day, in addition to meal times, in order to become comfortable with the procedure. The benefits you will get from this beginning practice will encourage more practice.

8. Act 2-Eat one meal using basic MMD food groups

Macronutrient composition.

Whenever you are going to prepare a meal, eat out or take out, you must be aware of the basic OGD food groups. The following fundamental food guidelines will get you started in the right direction. For healthy weight and longevity, our bodies are designed to work most efficiently and healthfully with a certain healthy combination and quantity of certain types of the macronutrients, carbohydrates, fats and proteins. The healthiest combination has been hotly debated and still is highly controversial due to the lack of long term studies to prove any particular concept. Basically popular diets have argued a certain ratio of each, which has varied over the years. As each diet plan attempts to claim market share, it grows and then fades due to lack of success and public interest wanes. The next new diet plan claims another ratio and goes through the same process. This has been going on for decades, as the ratio of macronutrients is being recycled to entice public interest. The OGD program breaks' this cycling of unsupported opinions by referencing the diets of the HALL peoples as the most credible healthy information presently available.

The basic micronutrient combinations of the HALL people is as follows

a. **CARBOHYDRATES** [carbs] – The majority of the HALL peoples diet is 55 to 65% carbohydrates, with the great majority in natural or complex carbs and a minimum of refined or simple carbs. Examples of natural include: unprocessed vegetables, fruits, and whole grains. The HALL peoples keep refined carbs to a minimum. Examples include refined and processed foods, such as white flour, sugar, soft drinks and bakery goods. The preference for natural carbs is also the case with virtually all US medical and health Organizations.

b. **FATS** –We are concerned with two basic types of fats. Those considered healthy are high in monounsaturated and polyunsaturated fats and are the HALL preference, as well as US health organizations. Fats considered 'unhealthy' are those high in saturated and/or trans fats. Recently the FDA, certain states and other health organizations have moved to virtually ban trans fats. The percentage of fat that can occur in a healthy diet depends on the degree and combination of 'healthy' and 'unhealthy' fats. If it is high in 'healthy' fats, such as: olive and canola oil, plant fats such as soy products, and nuts and seeds, up to 40% has been shown to be healthy. For instance, certain traditional healthy Mediterranean diets are up to 30-40% fat [mostly from olive oil]. On the other hand, certain Eastern Asian diets are in the 10 to 20% range of fats. To be more realistic about American tastes, OGD recommends a 20-30% healthy fat consumption. In any event, the 'unhealthy' saturated [red meats and full dairy] and trans fats [hydrogenated oils in processed foods], are minimally consumed by the HALL peoples, and should be limited to less than 7 %.of total calories. An optional minimum of low or no fat dairy, milk, yogurt, cheese, ice cream, etc. is acceptable.

c. **PROTEINS** – 10 to 15% of HALL diets is from high quality proteins [natural foods with minimal meat]. Such foods would include beans, fish, and low or no fat dairy,

OGD and HALL people food groups

Food	Servings	Frequency
Mostly whole grains [breads, pasta, cereals, brown rice, noodles]	7 or more	Daily
Vegetables	7 or more	Daily
Fruit	2 or more	Daily
Legumes [beans, peas]	2 or more	Daily
Dairy [low or nonfat skim milk, yogurt, cheese]	1-2	Daily
Animal meats/eggs/poultry	0-2	Weekly-optional
Fish – Salmon, trout, sardines	6-8 oz. total	Weekly
Other Omega-3 [flaxseed, soy products]	1	Daily
Nuts and seeds	1 oz. [1/3 c cup]	Daily
Olive oil [extra virgin]	1-2 tbl	Daily
Tea [green, black, oolong]	2 cups	Daily
Wine, beer, sake	Optional	1-2 drinks/day
Sweets	optional	rarely

9. ACT 3 - CONSUME 5-10% LESS CALORIES

To lose weight, short of surgical options, the bottom line is that you must consume fewer calories and/or expend more, no matter what the type of diet. It is no coincidence that the people of all of the countries that are healthier then the U.S. consume less calories. [except for certain Chinese communities]. As a result of food consumerism, American have gotten into the habit of consuming more calories than necessary, and the trend is increasing with the 'value' food marketing trend that seems to have no limit. One practical way to consume fewer calories is to develop a habit of eating 5 to 10% less at each meal. It doesn't seem like much, but over a period of time it can be very significant. This is almost accomplished automatically when you are eating mindfully, and are aware that you are about to eat. Since there is no realistic way to judge 5 to 10% less calories than normal, a practical way is to this is to make it a goal to leave the table just a little hungry, rather than with a feeling of being full. Ignore those last few mouthfuls you ordinarily would take. If you do this a few times, you will find that you feel more comfortable than being bloated. This becomes easier to do when you know, that if you need to, you can fill up later with fruits and vegetables.

Other techniques to consume fewer calories

1. Drinking water before meals will reduce appetite
2. Eat chunky rather than finely chopped salads and pureed soups to feel fuller.
3. Eat slowly to allow your satiety sensors to operate before you have overeaten. [They take about 20 minutes]
4. Eat foods high in unrefined carbohydrates and fiber to help keep calories low without a feeling of starvation. A sort of a 'eat more weigh less' strategy.
5. When overcooking the amounts recommended, use for another meal.
6. When eating at a restaurant, plan to take out a doggie bag, since the portion served will usually be a diet buster of unhealthy proportions.
7. If you are hungry for sweets, use natural sweets, such as ripe fruits.

10. ACT 4 - BURN AN EXTRA 100 CALORIES

A certain level of physical activity is essential not only to healthy weight loss but also to the state of energetic feeling and healthy longevity. Adequate levels of physical [and mental] activity are essential to meet a basic human design principle — 'use it or lose it'. A strong indication that nature designed us for certain levels of activity are displayed by the 'runners high', a well-known phenomenon that rewards exercise with pleasurable endorphins.

All of the HALL people were highly active, as compared to current American levels of activity. However, since most of these peoples worked hard all day in the fields, factories, or some other form of manual labor, it wasn't necessary to have fitness studios. Since most of us don't have the opportunity to physically work hard [that's what automation is all about – comfort without effort], guidelines practical for our culture that approximate the activity of the HALL are set forth in the OGD plan. For the initial one month plan, it's best to start out slow and build up a general liking for the good feeling that results from sensible exercise. For those who have been relatively inactive, a slower start will be easier to maintain, until the EMP program changes your thinking about physical activity. Regular physical activity also can help risk factors for several diseases and improve your overall health and feeling of wellbeing.

It does not matter what type of physical activity you perform—sports, planned exercise, household chores, yard work, or work-related tasks—all are beneficial, not only to weight loss but also general health. Studies show that even the most inactive people, at any age, can gain significant health benefits if they accumulate 30 minutes or more of physical activity per day. Substantial research consistently shows that regular physical activity, combined with healthy eating habits, is the most efficient and healthful way to control your weight.

Physical activity and weight

Physical activity helps to control your weight by using excess calories that otherwise would be stored as fat. Your body weight is regulated by the number of calories you eat and use each day. Virtually everything you eat and drink contains calories, and any energy you exert uses calories, including sleeping, breathing, and digesting food. Any physical activity in addition to what you normally does will use extra calories, and this is what makes increased activity so important in healthy weight loss.

Balancing the calories you use through physical activity with the calories you eat will help you achieve your desired weight. When you eat more calories than you need to perform your daily activities, your body stores the extra calories and you gain weight. Put simplistically, when you eat fewer calories than you use, your body uses the stored calories and you lose weight. When you eat the same amount of calories as your body uses, your weight stays the same. It doesn't exactly work this way because when you reduce your caloric input for a sufficient period of time, your body will make adjustments in your metabolic rate, appetite, etc. to try and prevent weight loss. This effect is common after two to three months on conventional diets, and is sometimes referred to as the plateau. However, the OGD diet is designed to help offset this process by preventing hunger, and by use of the Behavioral program to revise subconscious eating programs.

Any type of additional physical activity you choose to do—strenuous activities such as running or aerobic dancing or moderate-intensity activities such as walking or household work—will increase the number of calories your body uses. The key to successful weight control and improved overall health is developing the habit, so that physical activity a part of your daily routine. To start your physical activity program, select one of the activities from the Activity/Calorie table to burn an extra 100 calories per day.

11. ACTIVITY/CALORIES TABLE

**Approximate minutes it takes to burn
100 calories for different body weights**

ACTIVITY	125 lbs.	175 lbs.	225 lbs.
Bicycling, 6 mph	18	13	10
Bicycling, 12 mph	13	9	7
Bowling	35	25	20
Calisthenics	30	22	17
Dancing socially	16	12	9
Digging in the garden	21	15	12
Golf	23	17	13
Folding clothes	53	38	29

Jogging	15	11	8
Jumping rope	13	9	7
Mowing the lawn	19	14	11
Running in place	13	9	7
Running, 6 mph	11	8	6
Swimming, easy pace	18	13	10
Swimming, strenuous pace	13	9	7
Tennis, singles	15	11	7
Tennis, doubles	18	13	10
Walking, 2 mph	42	30	23
Walking, 3 mph	32	23	18
Vacuuming	30	22	17

Source, Mayo Clinic Health Letter, February 2003
FYI- To lose 1 pound a week by exercise, you need to burn 500 calories daily

12. DAILY ACTS JOURNAL

Now that you have reviewed the descriptions and instructions for the actions, it is now time to put the plan into effect. Journaling is a proven method to help create a habit. Daily recording the dates for the acts you have performed, will provide substantial support and acknowledgement of having met a goal. Don't be discouraged that you don't do all of the acts all of the time. This is the purpose of the MMD Behavioral program - to change your eating habits so that you will want to do them, and it will be automatic and you won't even have to think about it.

Key act- For this first month, practice mindfulness as frequently as you can, but at least once a day. It can be done virtually anytime you are waiting, walking, resting, etc. But not of course when your focus is demanded elsewhere, such as driving a car. The more mindful you are, the more you be in control of changing your eating habits, not to mention the additional benefits of less stress, worry and anxiety.

First month's MMD Behavioral plan - Weekly Journal

ACT	DESCRIPTION	FREQUENCY	DATE
1.	Practice mindful eating at one meal	One meal/day	
2.	Eat meal using OGD food groups	At least one/day	
3.	Eat 5-10% less at largest meal	At least one/day	
4.	Burn an extra 100 calories	Daily	

13. MONTH TWO - Changing eating habits

This program is designed to be used only after you have completed the one-month practice of the Month one 4 acts. Gaining more control of your mind by mindfulness is critical to make changes. The first month involved exercises for mindful eating, basic knowledge of healthy food types, calorie reduction, and physical activity. The next step is to change your habits for food preferences and eating patterns. Since we are creatures of habit, it is only by developing these habits that you will be able to sustain a long-term healthy weight. The main reason diets fail is because they attempt to use will power to overcome genetic food urges and unhealthy eating habits. Our 'sometimes' will power pitted against our genes or habits, working 24/7 is no contest. Just think about your New Year's Resolutions. Behavioral habits are generated by your subconscious mind. Unfortunately, your subconscious mind doesn't understand that the predisposition of your obesity genes, once essential for survival, is now unhealthy in today's environment. But fortunately your food preference is only a learned habit. Consequently, it can be changed, as shown by the common example of changing eating habits when relocating to another country

The goal of the EMP program is to adopt the basic food preferences of the HALL peoples, by changing eating habits. And while we can't change the predisposition of our 'obesity genes' for fat, sweets and overeating, we can substitute healthy fat, natural sweets and unlimited amounts of plant foods, just as these healthier peoples do. While initially, it appears unrealistic to think that you would prefer a tasty salad to a filet mignon that is precisely the eating habit change we are talking about. Speaking from personal experience, I was strictly a meat and while bread man for the first 40 years of my life. Southern fried chicken was considered a gourmet meal. Vegetables were considered food for our pet rabbits, and not something people would think of putting in their mouth. Then about 3 decades ago, I became aware of the continuing stream of studies linking animal products and heart disease. This coincided with Cooper's best seller 'Aerobics' promising that marathon runners developed immunity to heart disease, and I was converted. Within 6 months, my taste for animal products dissolved and vegetables, whole grain cereals and fish were my preferred foods, and I maintained my weight at 160 lbs. While one person's testimony may be interesting, it doesn't mean it's going to be applicable for others.

The reality is that most of the overweight don't have the will power to stop their march to obesity. They are being overpowered by their unhealthy innate eating habits, with the majority of Americans being forecast to be overweight within 15 years.

Since Behavioral habits' are linked to the subconscious region of our mind, it is necessary to communicate with our subconscious mind, which can only be done when the conscious mind can be bypassed. The most proven and effective of doing this is by hypnotherapy. The mind/body innovation of hypnotherapy is safe, effective and used in mainstream medicine for many other purposes, such as chronic pain and stress management and other forms of self-healing. In fact, we enter into the hypnotic state of mind on a daily basis when we engage in self-talk or daydreaming. In reality, hypnotherapy is nothing more than meditation with suggestions.

The EMP program is motivated by a combination of epigenetic innovations designed to change the way you think about eating and exercises. This program combines in a unique way, the exercise of mindfulness to put you more in control of your mind, the knowledge of how accomplish your goals, and hypnotherapy to change your eating habits.

14. Understanding EMP self-hypnosis

a. What is self-hypnosis?
b. your conscious and subconscious mind
c. Changing eating habits and reasons for eating
d. Install posthypnotic eating suggestions
e. Components of the EMP plan

The EMP mental conditioning program uses the principles of mindfulness, self-hypnosis and imaging in a program especially designed to encourage a healthy weight loss and its related healthy longevity. In this section the self-hypnosis and imaging components are described as mindfulness and mindful eating has already been described earlier in this chapter.

a. What is self-hypnosis?

Hypnosis is a form of a mind/body intervention that has many applications and is not easily defined-since it is a state of mind. It is frequently misunderstood as mysterious, but nothing could be further from the truth. Hypnosis simply is method of producing a deep state of relaxation where our subconscious is more receptive to suggestions. The main difference between meditation and hypnosis is that hypnosis facilitates the power of hypnotic suggestions. There are many levels of the hypnotic state, for instance you may experience driving down a highway, when all of a sudden you become aware that you have missed your turn, you were not driving irrationally and yet your mind was focused on something else. You actually were in a hypnotic state. Other examples include: daydreaming, reading a book, or watching TV. Even words can be hypnotic, and they can stimulate your imagination, creating a suggestive state in your mind. Meditation and prayer are also forms of a hypnotic state. In other words, at the time that you are doing something that you are not consciously thinking about you are under a state of hypnosis. .

Self-hypnosis is merely a self-induced form of hypnosis. You can apply self-hypnosis to virtually any activity or outcome that depends on your own efforts, or that you can influence with your mind. Sometimes it is so easy the results seem mysterious, and even miraculous, but it works in a consistent manner that can be explained, predicted and repeated. It's biology, not magic. In self-hypnosis, you are still in control and you will not do anything in a hypnotic state that you would not do while in a normal waking state.

b. Your conscious and unconscious mind

Your mind can be thought of as having two levels. Your conscious mind is the surface and your subconscious mind is the deep mental pool underneath. Einstein estimated that we work with no more than 10% of our mind. No wonder that the mind has been referred to as a "mental iceberg" since so much of its activity is below the surface and so much of its capacity is unused. Since your conscious mind makes up only about 10 percent of your total mind, as you become more practiced in self-hypnosis, you will find it easier to get information and energy from your subconscious mind. Your conscious mind is the communication center where you process thoughts and ideas. Here you think, calculate, plan, feel emotions and direct the outcome of your conscious actions. The conscious mind deals with all the information that enters it, both through the subconscious mind and through your external sensors of sight, hearing, touch, taste, and smell.

Our subconscious mind acts as our servant as far as habits is concerned. For instance, we learn at an early age to walk, eat our food with a knife and fork, to ride a bike, and prefer certain foods. The subconscious mind controls all the involuntary functions of the body such as digestion, breathing, heart rate, temperature, and so on. It is widely accepted that anxiety, stress and tension can negatively affect these function and the bad effects are known as psychosomatic illnesses. Since hypnosis can directly contact the subconscious mind, than hypnosis can bring about recovery. All our emotions are contained within the subconscious mind and since emotion is usually stronger then reason, our subconscious is frequently in charge. The subconscious mind contains our ability to use our imagination. And when you think about it worry is only a negative imagination. Our subconscious mind provides us with motivation; it directs our physical and emotional energy. For instance, if you decide to lose weight or some other goal, Most of the energy to make this change must come from the subconscious. Your unconscious mind is your storage center; it contains all the experiences you've had since birth. It also hosts your belief system, and acts as your conscious, sending you morally guiding messages about actions contemplated or performed. The subconscious mind is also responsible for your intuitive or gut feelings.

Some understanding is essential in making the most of self-hypnosis and suggestion... The conscious mind works to make changes in some situations, but subconscious oppositions often arises to block you from what you want, such as losing weight. The conscious mind says that being overweight is bad and losing weight is a good thing to do. But the subconscious will almost certainly be opposed to that change, as it is to any change. For the subconscious, overeating is important and it will not want to stop. The basic theme of the subconscious mind is self-interest and it wants that thing that are good for you, but what he subconscious considers good can actually be bad. What we consciously know to be good or bad does not have much influence on the subconscious.

Everything we learn at the subconscious level is the result of direct experience. The subconscious mind. does not philosophize or think logically. It will only accept what it directly experienced, which can also include that which is consciously imagined. We rely on that characteristic of the subconscious in suggestion application. Because of the subconscious way of dealing with "imagined experience", it harbors many beliefs, attitudes and values that are untrue. This is why you can simultaneously want and be two contradictory things. It is the reason a person can be overweight and want to be slender at the same time. In the subconscious, all time is now and there is no future or past. You are simultaneously a child, an adolescent and the present you. This is important for suggesting change.

Your subconscious does not appear to age and feels same through-out your life, which could explain why a traumatic incident in youth can last a lifetime Also the subconscious doesn't have to think to respond, and consequently is always faster than the conscious. This can easily result in sayings that you wish you hadn't made.

c. Changing eating habits and reasons for eating.

Considering the above, it is easy to see why we must work with our subconscious mind in order to make significant eating habit changes, as well as change unhealthy eating behavior for psycho-logical needs. Using EMP guided self-hypnosis; we focus the con-scious mind and use it to work with the subconscious in ways to meet our weight control goal. As previously discussed, in order to change our long term eating behavior, it is necessary to change our subconscious eating programs, and in particular, our food prefer-ence habit. Since these preferences are learned and not genetic, the behavioral change essentially is the same as changing a habit. Like most lifelong habits this is difficult if not impossible to do by will power alone, as attested to by the long term failure of virtually all conventional diet programs. The most practical mind/body intervention to accomplish this purpose is guided self-hypnosis and imaging scripts that are specially designed for this purpose. In addition, the EMP script employs posthypnotic suggestions, to correct unhealthy eating behaviors, such as those stemming from emotional and other psychological reasons.

d. Install posthypnotic eating suggestions

With sufficient practice, you will be able to give a posthypnotic suggestion during a hypnotic state that will exert itself later and under the conditions you stated. After sufficient practice, the use of posthypnotic suggestions can be very powerful. When you use only your willpower as most weight loss programs do, to change an eating behavior, you are only using about 10% of our mind. But if you can program your unconscious mind to change eating pat-tern, you now have 90% of your total mind to work with. And better yet, when you have a healthy subconscious program, its automatic, and you don't have to try and force yourself to eat healthy.

e. Understanding the components of EMP self-hypnosis plan

Goals - The first step is to formulate a specific definition of exactly what you want to accomplish. Saying you want to lose weight may make conscious sense, but such simple goal formulations won't get you very far with the subconscious mind. To have any influence with the subconscious mind, goals must be clear and unambiguous. When you are formulating your suggestions it is necessary to know the specific behaviors you must develop to achieve your goal. For example, to reach your weight loss goal, you might set a weight loss of 2 pounds/ per week. The behaviors necessary to reach that goal, would be to learn the diets and lifestyles described in the MMD plan, practice mindful eating for one meal a day, and burn an extra 100 calories a day

Suggestions - The power of suggestion has a substantial influence on our behavior, beliefs, attitudes and values. We are wired to continually monitor information coming to us through the five senses, always on the lookout for opportunity and especially at the subconscious level, on guard against threat. Much of the information that is important to us is suggestive in nature. In short we are built to respond to suggestion. The suggestions we are talking about don't suggest a voluntary response but rather a hypnotic suggestion that will produce a non-voluntary response. The effectiveness of suggestion has been demonstrated over and over again in every field of medicine and human behavior. A prime example is the use of placebos. To get the placebo effect, one must know that they are being treated and that an increase in suggestion will produce an increase in placebo effect. Advertising is an excellent example of the practical application of suggestion. Most people say that advertising does not affect them but it is working on someone because sales go up when advertising is increased. To illustrate how suggestion lays a role in almost all areas of behavior consider Pavlov dogs. When he ran a bell the dogs would salivate. He had discovered classical conditioning, which is a conditioned response to suggestion. We all have our own equivalent of Pavlov's bell.

In self hypnosis, suggestions are one more way to the subconscious mind... But while we are sensitive to the power of suggestion, the primary function of our subconscious is to protest us, and consequently will reject suggestions that it perceives to be threatening or not in your best interest. For example, if you subconsciously believe that meat is necessary for better health, then a suggestion to change your eating preference to plant foods will not be effective.

Suggestions include affirmations and can be verbal or silent or an image. The OGD plan, recommends silent verbal and image suggestions. Of these two, image suggestions are usually easier and tend to be generally more effective then verbal. The reason for this is that the subconscious mind is far better at working with images then language, as demonstrated by dreams being almost entirely visual. The subconscious is designed to primarily communicate by imagery and emotion, with emotions presenting a power force in suggestions. For this reason, even when you are not in a hypnotic state, images or ideas about yourself and your place in the world, particularly backed by emotions, increase their likelihood of coming true. Consequently don't say negative things about yourself, because you increase their chances of coming true by the power of suggestion. Rather, although it sounds oversimplified, think you are happy and you will more likely to be happy and consciously keeping a half smile is a positive reminder. While is true that to make a habit change in the subconscious repetition of the suggestion is necessary, the reverse effect can be encountered if one tries too hard. Insomniacs experience this when they try to force themselves to sleep. Work with the subconscious must be done in a state of relaxation rather than under stressful conditions.

Emotions - Emotions must often be dealt with to achieve a goal. Emotion is the opposite of reason, in conscious terms. It includes all those things we feel; like love, hate, desire, fear, anger, disgust, grief, surprise and joy. In general if it something you feel and you did not arrive at by way of logic or reason, it is an emotion. To reduce a negative emotion, focus on eliminating it's most common symptom – 'the flight or fight syndrome' of rapid breathing, racing heart, etc., by returning to the breathing exercises discussed under Mindfulness and Breath control.

Guidelines for Verbal Suggestions - Suggestions must be clear, precise, and simple. For example the suggestion "Every day, in every way, I am getting better and better" would be too not specific and likely ineffective. Concrete words that refer to things that can be seen and touched. are the best for suggestions, such as in the following guidelines.

- Keep it personal. Use I instead of you, or say "I am" instead of "it is"
- Use a positive formulation. A positive formulation is better than a negative. Emphasize what you are going to do rather than what you are not going to do. For example "I prefer vegetables" is better than "I do not avoid vegetables"
- Timing and tense - Timing is an important factor. Use "I am" rather than "I am becoming" The reason is the subconscious mind has no sense of past and future. Exception to this can be taken when it is a suggestion that is to take place at a particular time or event, such as when sitting down to a meal. .

Suggestion -examples

- The Western diet is a risk factor for cardiovascular diseases and cancer
- Animal fat gives heart disease
- Plant foods make you healthier and longer lived.
- People that eat large steaks are fat and unhealthy
- Thin people are healthier and have fewer disabilities
- Fat people are unattractive
- I am losing 1 lb. per week
- I am burning an extra 100 calories a day
- I am getting thinner and healthier.

Image Suggestion Formulation - Image suggestion are composed of pictures instead of words and more effective then verbal suggestions. Likewise, imagination is more powerful that language. The focus of an image suggestion should be a graphic representation of one or more goals or objective. Begin with a verbal suggestion around which you can construct the images need for image constructions. For example with the suggestion 'I am burning an extra 100 calories a day', imagine yourself physically doing some type of exercise, such as walking or climbing a flight of stairs. As another example of the suggestion 'I prefer to eat vegetables rather than meat', form an image in your 'mind's eye' of pushing away a hamburger, in favor of a bowl of tasty salad. Make this as vivid as you can, such as your taste rejection of the hamburger and the tasty appeal of the salad.

Image suggestions can have different meaning attached to them, such as; intellectual, emotional, and physical. An intellectual meaning is what you think and the way you would describe it to someone else. The emotional meaning strengths the intellectual meaning and makes it more effective. For instance, expecting to feel good improves the likelihood of actually feeling good. The physical meaning relates to your body and its senses. For instance, imagine a particular pain going away. Metaphors work well in image suggestions. An example of a metaphor is an image of you floating peacefully and serenely on calm water, in which the suggestion is of self-control and calmness. Metaphors dispense with the connecting words and instead do their job by familiar comparisons. Visual imagery has been clinically shown to be beneficial with many diseases, such as cancer, arthritis, high blood pressure, and many more. Since it I is impossible to know every process involved in a healing, simplified metaphor are used. Attack visualizations are a kind of metaphor that can be effective, such as a cancer tumor being eaten by a killer cell. You don't have to limit your suggestions to just when you are practicing self-hypnosis. You can repeat your suggestions while you are engaged in other activities, as long it will not distract you from something that requires your full attention.

When do suggestions become effective - If you don't see at least some results by the end of three weeks, reexamine your suggestions, looking for something that is blocking the process. When you do see some positive changes, don't assume that they are from changes due to natural causes and not the suggestion. Discontinuing your suggestion too soon can result in the unwanted condition returning. This is not uncommon, since changes that occur as the result of suggestion will almost always feel natural and effortless. With image suggestions, it is more a matter of duration then number of repetitions. The longer you hold an image in your mind the more it is likely to become a reality, however, 10 to 15 seconds, several times a day is generally effective. Bedtime is an excellent time to apply your suggestions. Just before going to sleep, repeat your verbal suggestions or visualize your image suggestions. This has a way of loading them into the subconscious mind which will work with them while you are asleep.

The most powerful tool in self-hypnosis is the posthypnotic suggestion. When in a hypnotic state the conscious mind loses its ability to make critical decisions, and during that time your subconscious can accept the suggestion as a reality. A powerful suggestion continues to function after the hypnotic state has ended and your conscious mind accepts your suggestion as part of its decision making process. The deeper the hypnotic state, the easier it is to implant the suggestion into your subconscious mind. The more you experience the suggestion as a reality the more it will actually be a reality in your waking state. Suggestions are very powerful methods to change the habits in your subconscious mind. In the OGD program, your suggestions under hypnosis become active after the hypnosis state is ended, when triggered by a prearranged word or act.

What we are and how we react to events and to other people is all dictated by earlier life programming. The first way we can look at reprogramming is through affirmations or talking to ourselves. We all talk to ourselves a lot of the time and this inner dialogue is powerful stuff. So powerful that it can affect everything what we say or do. If while in hypnosis you repeat the simple affirmation in your mind, "I am getting slimmer" you can change the way you think about yourself. It sounds overly simple, but remembers that in hypnosis you talk directly to your subconscious mind and if you repeat the affirmation enough, your mind will eventually believe it. The subconscious mind is like a child and cannot comprehend long intellectual phrases, so keep your affirmations simple and emotional. For example 'I am going to have a healthy weight and feel good'

Imagery – Another way we can look at mental programming is through the mind/body intervention of self-guided imagery. In hypnosis you have direct access to your subconscious mind of which a part is your imagination. Using your imagination in hypnosis can be very powerful. Suppose you are overweight, and you see yourself as being fat every time you look in the mirror. You see yourself as fat whenever you think about yourself and you desperately want to lose weight. But however many diets you go on, however much you deprive yourself of food, you still know that you are fat. That image of yourself is well embedded into your mind and effects your perception of yourself. Using imaging, when you take yourself into hypnosis you can give your subconscious mind a positive image of the way you want to be. Using positive affirmations, your subconscious mind soon gets the message and starts having different ideas about the 'slimmer you' that is within you. Add to the positive affirmation, an image of yourself becoming slimmer, such as used in the EMP self-hypnosis induction script.

Suggestion triggers - A trigger produces a reaction to a posthypnotic suggestion that was planted in your subconscious mind during a self-hypnotic state. It may be a word or a touch, a sound or a visual cue, a smell or a taste, or an emotion. The stronger the suggestion that you implanted, the greater effect the trigger has in recreating the response. You can then create a posthypnotic suggestion to respond to a positive trigger that you implanted in your own subconscious mind. When are practicing a hypnotic induction, and you reach zero, tell yourself that you will feel very comfortable in a favorite place in your mind that is calm and relaxing.

This place may be from your memory, a new place or just a place deep inside yourself, where you can have positive experiences. Beautiful places in nature, such as gardens and ocean beaches have wide appeal. Once you have entered a hypnotic state, tell yourself to place your thumb and forefinger together [or your preferred word or touch that is meaningful to you]. This will be your trigger, and it will remind you of how relaxed and calm you were feeling at that moment. Every time you practice self-hypnosis and reinforce your trigger it will become stronger and stronger in your subconscious mind. Each time you trigger your suggestion it will work better and be more responsive. Your trigger is also used to initiate other posthypnotic suggestions, as described in the self-hypnosis script.

15. Self-Hypnosis Induction Procedure

For your first few self-hypnosis practices perform the Relaxation and Deeping exercises to condition your mind for the change of mental state.

Relaxation Response

The first step and most critical in communicating with your subconscious is to enter a state of relaxation. For purposes of self-hypnosis, the following exercise is most practical and user friendly. It is a genetic reaction called 'The Relaxation Response' and consequently works naturally with all people. Consequently, it is used in mainstream medicine, and recommended by the National Institutes of Health. Practice it a few times to get some experience. You will notice that key words are used over and over. This is important since suggestion is greatly heightened in a hypnotic state. . 'Relax' is one of them, repeat it slowly and feel relaxed while you are saying it. If you were to mentally say the word 'heavy' you might feel heaviness and similarly for 'lighter' and 'deeper'. Imaging what these words feel and look like strengthens the suggestion. When you come back to normal consciousness, feel refreshed in your mind and body.

First make yourself as comfortable as possible you may sit or lie down. Take a breath of air, fill your lungs to a comfortable level and focus on an object in front of you, slowly exhaling your breath, and then fill your lungs again. Slowly let your eyes go out of focus, as you continue breathing in this slow manner, and imagine releasing the tension in your muscles. Start progressively relaxing the muscles throughout your entire body in an orderly sequence, such as; first feel your feet relaxing, then feel the tension going out of the muscles in your lower legs and continuing to relax the muscles in your lower body, and progressing through your chest, arms, and neck. How long this process should take and the muscle detail is a personal choice that works best for you.

Deepening Techniques - called deepening because it deepens both the relaxation and the hypnotic trance state. Of the many deepening techniques, the most popular involves counting backward. The EMP program starts at 5 and slowly count downward toward zero, imaging relaxing more deeply with each number. This state of increasing relaxation is similar to going to sleep, except that you continue to be aware. It is important to use your imagination during this phase. For example, imagine that you are on an elevator while counting down, and that each number is a different floor level and you see each floor number lighting up as you move downward. The last stop is zero where you reach your 'favorite place.' As you continue to count down, imaging yourself becoming more and more relaxed.

The deeper the hypnosis the more relaxed you become. After you have practiced self-hypnosis a few times, you may be interested in going to a deeper level to get more power in your suggestions and affirmations in changing your eating habits and eating behavior. Once you have relaxed to a state where you are on your favorite place [garden bench, beach, nature setting, etc.] Try the examples below to determine which works best for you.

1. Raise your right arm a few inches up into the air and as you drop it heavily back into your lap, give yourself the suggestion that you will take yourself three times deeper. Just decide to let it happen.
2. Take a long deep breath and as you breathe out, give yourself the suggestion that you will take yourself three times deeper.
3. Just say to yourself the word "deeper" two or three times, telling yourself that you will take yourself deeper each time you say the word.
4. Imagine that you are walking slowly down a very long staircase and tell yourself that each step you take takes you deeper into hypnosis.
5. Any other visualizations or imaging that you can focus on that brings more relaxation.

15. EMP SELF HYPNOSIS SCRIPT

General

The procedures recommended by this script or its associated CD must be practiced to become effective. Like any program to modify behavior, some repetition is necessary. The practice required for this program to help you change your life is individualistic, depending on various personal circumstances. However, the program uses epigenetic influences that have been shown in studies to be effective and generally applicable. In other words, what you get out of it will be in proportion to what you put into it. If you perform the exercises in this chapter, faithfully and purposely, chances are good that it will work for you in changing your eating habits.

Time limits

We usually have a restricted time to perform the exercises, and you may be concerned that you will fall asleep. After sufficient practice, in order to restrict any occasion on which you may fall asleep, as you enter the hypnosis state, say 'hypnosis now for five minutes' or whatever time limit you want. You will not need to awaken yourself consciously this time by counting backwards from five to zero; your subconscious mind will automatically do that for you.

Procedure

The lines in bold are yours or a guide instructor. If self-administered, say them silently to yourself. The suggested timing [i.e. wait 2 sec or just 2 sec] can be modified to suit individual preferences. Get yourself in comfortable sitting position, where you won't be disturbed.

Close your eyes and perform the breathing exercise you practiced for mindful eating, in ACT 1. Focus on your breathing, feel your breath coming in your left nostril and then out your right nostril. Breathing normally and be conscious to your breathing......

Breathe in to the count of 1 and out to the count of 2, [2sec]

In to the count of 3 and out to the count of 4 [2sec]

In to the count of 5 and out to the count of 6. [2sec]

In to the count of 7 and out to the count of 8, [2sec]

In to the count of 9 and out to the count of 10. [2sec]

I will stop while you repeat this breathing exercise yourself [stops for 15 seconds]

Now stop your counting and concentrate on my voice, while you continue your Rhythmic breathing.

Invite your body to release any tension, and imagine the tension is melting away as you focus on each part of the body.

Invite your feet and ankles to relax and notice how they respond, [wait 2 sec]

Imagine your legs are completely relaxed. [wait 2 sec]

Now feel the tension melt out of your hips [wait 2 sec]

Feel the tension dissolve in your body as you feel your abdomen relax

Now feel the softness flow up from your abdomen up to your chest; relax [2 sec]

Now feel your arms relax and become soft [wait 2 sec]

Finally imagine all the tension dissolves from your neck, so that your whole body is relaxed, and all the stress and tension has dissolved. You are now in a deep state of relaxation [wait 3 sec.]

In a moment you will count down from 5 and you will imagine your favorite place, it can be anywhere that is very beautiful and private, where you feel so relaxed and peaceful. [wait 3 sec]

It could be in a beautiful garden, where you can smell the wonderful aromas wafting on the light breeze, while you feel warmed by the sun and alone with the beauty of nature. [wait 3 sec]

Or it could be on a sandy beach with the blue waves breaking on the shore and the sandpipers skirting the changing water edge. And you can smell the aromas and hear the sounds of the surf and feel the sand between your toes. [wait 2 sec]

Now we start to count down to get to your favorite place

5- And you relax deeper

4-You are feeling more peaceful

3-Feel how comfortable you are - soon you will be in your favorite place

2 - Your breathing is regular and

1 - You are almost there

0 - It is so good to be here [2 sec]

You are so glad to be in your favorite place where you are so relaxed and have not a care in the world. Take some time to use all your senses to fully imagine your favorite place. You may hear the sounds and smell the aromas or even imagine a favorite taste. [5 sec]

Listen to my voice and believe the suggestions I am going to give you will make you slimmer and healthier and you will enjoy life so much more. You will follow them without effort.

Imagine the disadvantages of your present unhealthy eating and exercise habits. [2 sec]
See how they are making you overweight and threatening your health. [2 sec]
Image how your overweight makes you look to others. [2 sec]
Image all the energy it takes to drag around all that unhealthy fat. [2 sec]
You can almost feel the chest pains as your arteries become more and more plugged with animal fat. [2 sec]
Now image how being slim will make you look. [2 sec]
Image that you are feeling healthier and more energetic. [2 sec]
Image being able to fit into clothes you can't wear any more. [2 sec]
Imaging how your relationships will get better. [2 sec]

You want to get rid of the unhealthy habits of eating foods that make you overweight ... disease prone ....and decrease your quality of life, but you are unable to break these habits. You have been unable to break your unhealthy eating habits because they are rooted in your genes and childhood environment. But you believe that you can break unhealthy eating habits by replacing them with healthy ones.

Now imagine your present self as a **dark outline** of an overweight figure projected on a screen. ......Now imagine your new self as a thinner white outline overlaying the dark outline.
Imagine the new white outline is becoming slimmer ....and slimmer until you cover less .....and less of the dark outline you used to be. Whenever you think of the words '**SLIM FIGURE**' you will see this image in your mind's eye.

Now repeat the following affirmations, after me. [2 sec after each]
I can change my food preference because it is only a habit
I can satisfy my obesity genes with healthy fats, natural sweets and plant foods.

I will lose weight and be healthier eating mostly fruits, vegetables and whole grains

I will practice mindful eating, so I don't eat unhealthy or emotionally...

Overeating is an unhealthy habit and I will practice eating fewer calories

I am not worried about being hungry because I know I can always eat unlimited plant foods.

I know that more exercise will make me healthier and more energetic

I enjoy food, but I am not interested in more than needed for good health and nutrition.

I am feeling better and better as I become satisfied eating less.

I eat for good health, not to try to solve emotional problems or for comfort.

Food is not a substitute for love or attention.

When I eat healthy foods and exercise more I have more energy and feel better.

As I become thinner, I enjoy life more and more and feel alert and alive.

Now is the time to implant in your subconscious healthy eating suggesting which will remain with you after you have awakened.
    Repeat after me
If I crave unhealthy foods, I will put my hand on my stomach and think '**SLIM FIGURE**' imagining the thinner outline of my white figure against my old larger dark figure.

If I feel hungry at an inappropriate time I will place my hand on my stomach and think the words '**SLIM FIGURE**' and imagine my white figure outline.

Now let the image of your favorite place fade, as you come up to the surface of your mind as I count up to five. [2sec]
You will feel calm and relaxed as you know you can return whenever you want.

Zero – become aware of your breathing

One – If you crave unhealthy animal based food, you will place your hand over your stomach and think '**SLIM FIGURE**'

Two – You are coming back to the surface and will become mindful

Three – Whenever you are thinking about food, you will imagine your 'white **SLIM FIGURE**' overshadowed by your larger former dark figure outline.

Four – Whenever you think about your favorite place you will think about your food preference for natural plant foods.

Five – Take a deep breath, inhaling deeply and exhaling, as you have returned to the surface of your mind. You are fully awake and refreshed. Take a moment to adjust to your surroundings with a brief mindful breathing exercise counting up to 10 [wait 4 sec], The more you practice this induction, the sooner you will develop the new eating and exercise habits that will lead to a slimmer and healthier figure for life.

This procedure should be initially practiced daily for at least 5 minutes using this script or a guide, until your new eating habits become automatic, and you have lost significant weight. Your practice should be journalized to provide motivational support.

CHAPTER SEVEN

Physical activity
and weight control

1. How physical Activity helps control weight.
2. The Health Benefits of physical activity
3. The right amount of physical activity
4. Moderate-intensity activity
5. Aerobic activity
6. Stretching and Muscle Strengthening Exercises
7. Tips to a safe and successful physical activity program

1. How physical activity helps control weight

Physical activity helps to control your weight by using excess calories that otherwise would be stored as fat. Your body weight is regulated by the number of calories you eat and use each day. Everything you eat contains calories, and everything you do uses calories, including sleeping, breathing, and digesting food. Any physical activity in addition to what you normally does will use extra calories, and this is what makes increases activity so important in healthy weight loss.

Balancing the calories you use through physical activity with the calories you eat will help you achieve your desired weight. When you eat more calories than you need to perform your day's activities, your body stores the extra calories and you gain weight. Put simplistically, when you eat fewer calories than you use, your body uses the stored calories and you lose weight. When you eat the same amount of calories as your body uses, your weight stays the same. It doesn't work quite this simply, because when you reduce your caloric input for a sufficient period of time, your body will make adjustments in your metabolic rate, appetite, etc. to try and prevent it. However, MMD diet is designed to help offset this process by preventing hunger.

Any type of physical activity you choose to do–strenuous activities such as running or aerobic dancing or moderate-intensity activities such as walking or household work–will increase the number of calories your body uses. The key to successful weight control and improved overall health is making physical activity a part of your daily routine

To give you a feeling for the minutes in certain activities necessary to burn 100 calories, for different body weight, refer to the following table

Approximate minutes it takes to burn 100 calories

ACTIVITY	125 lbs.	175 lbs.	225 lbs.
Bicycling, 6 mph	18	13	10
Bicycling, 12 mph	13	9	7
Bowling	35	25	20
Calisthenics	30	22	17
Dancing socially	16	12	9
Digging in the garden	21	15	12
Golf	23	17	13
Folding clothes	53	38	29
Jogging	15	11	8
Jumping rope	13	9	7
Mowing the lawn	19	14	11
Running in place	13	9	7

Running, 6 mph	11	8	6
Sleeping	117	84	65
Standing	53	38	29
Swimming, easy pace	18	13	10
Swimming, strenuous pace	13	9	7
Tennis, singles	15	11	7
Tennis, doubles	18	13	10
Walking, 2 mph	42	30	23
Walking, 3 mph	32	23	18
Vacuuming	30	22	17

alth Letter, February 2003

To lose 1 pound a week by physical activity, you need to burn 500 calories a day.

2. The Health benefits of physical activity

In addition to helping to control your weight, research show that regular physical activity can reduce your risk for several diseases and conditions and improve your overall quality of life. Regular physical activity can help protect you from the following.

- Heart Disease and Stroke. Daily physical activity can help prevent heart disease and stroke by strengthening your heart muscle, lowering your blood pressure, raising your high density lipoprotein [HDL] levels [good cholesterol] and lowering low-density lipoprotein [LDL] levels [bad cholesterol], improving blood flow, and increasing your headrest's working capacity
- High Blood Pressure. Regular physical activity can reduce blood pressure I those with high blood pressure levels. Physical activity also reduces body fatness,
- Noninsulin-Dependent Diabetes. By reducing body fatness, physical activity can help to prevent and control this type of diabetes.

- Obesity. Physical activity helps to reduce body fat by building or preserving muscle mass and improving the body's ability to use calories. When physical activity is combined with proper nutrition, it can help control weight and prevent obesity, a major risk factor for many diseases.
- Back Pain. By increasing muscle strength and endurance and improving flexibility and posture, regular exercise helps to prevent back pain.
- Osteoporosis. Regular weight −bearing exercise promotes bone formation and may prevent many forms of bone loss associated with aging

Studies on the psychological effects of exercise have found that regular exercise increases your energy level, as well as an excellent method of stress reduction. Researchers also have found that exercise in likely to reduce depression and anxiety and help; you to manage stress.

3. The right amount of exercise.

If you are virtually inactive, a walk, tailored to your physical fitness more than any additional physical activity is beneficial. If you are already somewhat active, such that you can do any of the activities on the burn 100 calories chart, the more exercise you get the better. All the physical activities can be best measured by calories burned. Landmark studies of large groups of men [the Harvard Alumni Study] and women [The Nurse Study] suggest that those who burn an extra 700 or more calories a week by a dynamic exercise have healthier longevities than those who aren't as active. The type of exercises performed in these studies where intensive enough to increase heart and breathing rate significantly. These studies also seemed to indicate that over 2,000 calories a week [walking about 3 miles a day] the health benefits leveled out. However, from a weight loss perspective, the more calories you burn, the more weight you lose.

For the greatest overall health benefits, experts recommend that you do 20 to 30 minutes of aerobic activity three or more times a week and some type of muscle strengthening activity and stretching at least twice a week. However, if you are unable to do this level of activity, you can gain substantial health benefits by accumulating 30 minutes or more of moderate-intensity physical activity a day, at least five times a week. If you have been inactive for a while, you may want to start with less strenuous activities such as walking or swimming at a comfortable pace. Beginning at a slow pace will allow you to become physically fit without straining your body. Once you are in better shape, you can gradually do more strenuous activity.

4. Moderate intensity activity

Moderate-intensity activities include some of the things you may already be doing during a day or week, such as gardening and housework. These activities can be done in short spurts–10 minutes here, 8 minutes there. Alone, each action does not have a great effect on your health, but regularly accumulating 30 minutes of activity over the course of the day can result in substantial healthy weight loss and health benefits.

To become more active throughout your day, take advantage of any chance to get up and move around. Here are some examples:

- Take a short walk around the block
- Rake leaves
- Play actively with the kids
- Walk up the stairs instead of taking the elevator
- Mow the lawn
- Take an activity break–get up and stretch or walk around
- Park your car a little farther away from your destination and walk the extra distance.

The point is not to make physical activity an unwelcome chore, but to make the most of the opportunities you have to be active.

5. Aerobic activity

Aerobic activity is an important addition to moderate-intensity exercise. Aerobic exercise is any extended activity that makes you breathe hard while using the large muscle groups at a regular, even pace. Aerobic activities help make your heart stronger and more efficient. They also use more calories and consequently more weight loss, than other activities. Some examples of aerobic activities include:

- Brisk walking
- Jogging
- Bicycling
- Swimming
- Aerobic dancing
- Racket sports
- Rowing
- Ice or roller skating
- Cross-country or downhill skiing
- Using aerobic equipment (i.e., treadmill, stationary bike)

To get the most health benefits from aerobic activity, you should exercise at a level strenuous enough to raise your heart rate to your target zone. Your target heart rate zone is 50 to 75 percent of your maximum heart rate (the fastest your heart can beat). To find your target zone, look for the category closest to your age in the chart below and read across the line. For example, if you are 35 years old, your target heart rate zone is 93-138 beats per minute.

Age	Target Heart Rate Zone 50-75%	Average Maximum Heart Rate 100%
20-30 years	98-146 beats per min.	195
31-40 years	93-138 beats per min.	185
41-50 years	88-131 beats per min.	175
51-60 years	83-123 beats per min.	165
61+ years	78-116 beats per min	155

To see if you are exercising within your target heart rate zone, count the number of pulse beats at your wrist or neck for 15 seconds, then multiply by four to get the beats per minute. Your heart should be beating within your target heart rate zone. If your heart is beating faster than your target heart rate, you are exercising too hard and should slow down. If your heart is beating slower than your target heart rate, you should exercise a little harder. When you begin your exercise program, aim for the lower part of your target zone (50 percent). As you get into better shape, slowly build up to the higher part of your target zone (75 percent). If exercising within your target zone seems too hard, exercise at a pace that is comfortable for you. You will find that, with time, you will feel more comfortable exercising and can slowly increase to your target zone.

6. Stretching and muscle strengthening exercises

While the physical activity is often the only exercise recommended for weight loss, strength training should be part of any overall exercise program. At about age 45, muscle mass begins to decline at a rate of about 1 percent a year. And as muscle mass decreases, so does muscle strength. And as strength goes, so can the ability to perform the physical activity necessary for weight maintenance. A deterioration of strength also affects the overall quality of life, such as the ability to climb stairs, do chores, dance, take walks, go grocery shopping or accomplish other daily activities. Muscle loss occurs in people of all fitness levels, even outstanding athletes. But those who have less muscle to begin with pay a higher price. As strength deteriorates, to a point where it is uncomfortable to perform daily tasks, people shy away from them, and the reduction in using the muscles, further weakens them. While it is common knowledge that strength training, such as weight lifting and resistance machines increases muscle mass in younger people, it is less known to the public that the same response, is true with older people. However, many recent studies have shown that strength for training for older people is also highly effective. In one study men ranging in age from 60 to 72 more than doubled their leg strength in just 12 weeks of strength training, and in another study frail nursing home residents in their 90s where demonstrated to build muscle and strength.

The way strength training works is that sufficient straining of muscles causes microscopic tears in those muscles, which the muscles rebuild protein in those cells, making them stronger. Consequently, it shouldn't be done two days in a row, to allow the muscles sufficient time to rebuild from the strain, and two to three workouts a week is sufficient. Your program should be done initially with a qualified personal trainer to get the knowledge for the most effect training for a person your age and physical condition. Typically a workout might consist of 6 to 8 different types of exercises or resistances on a progress basis that will allow you to do about 6 repetitions for each type of exercise before it becomes too uncomfortable. After it becomes easy to 6 reps, then the reps can be increased on subsequent sessions until you can do 10. After several workouts and 10 reps only requires a minimum strain, and then increase the weight, until you can only do 6 repetitions and start the process over. The exercises should be selected to fully include your body and only concentrated on a certain part of the body for a particular goal, such a particularly weak part. It is generally recommended that you get your doctor's OK before your start, just in case your health condition might limit your exercise

Stretching muscles

While stretching is not high on the list of burning calories it helps condition our body, so that we are better prepared for exercise. Stretching comes naturally to all of us. If we have been sitting in a particular position for a long time, we stretch unconsciously. Stretching has many benefits; such as reducing muscle tension, increases range of joints, helps to prepare the body for physical activity, helps prevent injuries, increases blood circulation, and enhances muscular co-ordination. The basic principles of stretching are simple. The stretch should be held for 10-20 seconds for each muscle group, and done without any bouncy movements. Breathing should be rhythmic, slow and under control. Do not hold your breath during exercise. Many of the stretches are well known and instinctive. Various types are readily available in exercise media and on line. Information on types of yoga, Tai Chi and other movements are helpful in stretching as well as general wellbeing, are readily available.

7. Tips for a safe and successful physical activity program

Make sure you are in good health. Answer the following questions* before you begin exercising.

1. Has a doctor ever said you have heart problems?
2. Do you frequently suffer from chest pains?
3. Do you often feel faint or have dizzy spells?
4. Has a doctor ever said you have high blood pressure?
5. Has a doctor ever told you that you have a bone or joint problem, such as arthritis, that has been or could be aggravated by exercise?
6. Are you over the age of 65 and not accustomed to exercise?
7. Are you taking prescription medications, such as those for high blood pressure?
8. Is there a good medical reason, not mentioned here, why you should not exercise?

If you answered "yes" to any of these questions, you should see your doctor before you begin an exercise program.

- Follow a gradual approach to exercise to get the most benefits with the fewest risks. If you have not been exercising, start at a slow pace and as you become fit, gradually increase the amount of time and the pace of your activity.

- Choose activities that you enjoy and that fit your personality. For example, if you like team sports or group activities; choose things such as soccer or aerobics. If you prefer individual activities, choose things such as swimming or walking. Also, plan your activities for a time of day that suits your personality. If you are a morning person, exercise before you begin the rest of your day's activities. If you have more energy in the evening, plan activities that can be done at the end of the day. You will be more likely to stick to a physical activity program if it is convenient and enjoyable.

- Exercise regularly. To gain the most health benefits it is important to exercise as regularly as possible. Make sure you choose activities that will fit into your schedule.

- Exercise at a comfortable pace. For example, while jogging or walking briskly you should be able to hold a conversation. If you do not feel normal again within 10 minutes following exercise, you are exercising too hard. Also, if you have difficulty breathing or feel faint or weak during or after exercise, you are exercising too hard.

- Maximize your safety and comfort. Wear shoes that fit and clothes that move with you, and always exercise in a safe location. Many people walk in indoor shopping malls for exercise. Malls are climate controlled and offer protection from bad weather.

- Vary your activities. Choose a variety of activities so you don't get bored with any one thing.

- Encourage your family or friends to support you and join you in your activity. If you have children, it is best to build healthy habits when they are young. When parents are active, children are more likely to be active and stay active for the rest of their lives.

- Challenge yourself. Set short-term as well as long-term goals and celebrate every success, no matter how small.

Whether your goal is to control your weight or just to feel healthier, becoming physically active is a step in the right direction. Take advantage of the health benefits that regular exercise can offer and make physical activity a part of your lifestyle. Remember the cardinal rule of our human design −'Use it or lose it'

Weight loss and intensity of exercise

For many years, the "no pain, no gain" school has held sway in many areas, including weight loss. The concept being that a higher duration an intensity of exercise may improve long-term weight loss. . This concept has been disproved according to a study published in the September 10, 2003 edition of the Journal of the American Medical Association. The randomized trial was performed on almost 201 women who were normally sedentary, overweight, had a mean age of 37 and a mean body mass index of 32.6. The women were assigned to one of four groups -moderate or vigorous intensity with high duration and moderate or vigorous intensity with moderate duration. The exercise intensity was designed to burn either 1,000 or 2,000 calories a week for 12 months.

All women were instructed to reduce intake of energy between 1200 and 1500 kcal/d and dietary fat to between 20 to 30% of total energy intake. All women lost 8 to 12 percent of their weight and maintained most of the weight loss. There were no significant differences among the four groups. The women who walked at least 40 minutes a day lost significantly more weight than those who walked less than 30 minutes daily. But even those who walked the least maintained a 6 percent weight loss. More than 9 out of 10 stayed with the exercise plan.

APPENDIX A

Recommended good groups

DAILY FOOD CHOICES at a Glance

Preferred Unprocessed Foods	Servings	Frequency
Vegetables of wide variety	7 - 13	Per day
Grains- mostly whole - bread, rice, noodles, cereals	7-13	Per day
Fruit - wide variety	2-4	Per day
Flavonoid Foods [i.e. - soy products, flaxseed, miso, tea, etc.]	2-4	Per day
Calcium Foods - [i.e. -skim milk, green leafy vegetables, soy milk and beans]	2-4	Per day
Omega -3 Foods [i.e.-fatty fish, flaxseed, etc.]	1-3	Per day
Olive oil	1-2 tbl	Per day
Meat, Poultry and eggs	0-7	Per Week
Sweets	0-3	Per Week
Tea [i.e.- black, green, oolong]	1-3	Daily

1. Eat a variety of foods, the majority from plant sources. Number of servings dependent on calorie requirements.
2. About 55% to 65% of diet to be carbohydrates [the great majority to be complex   minimize simple carbohydrate intake such as sugar, processed and bakery foods.] 20 to 30

% from fats [the majority from olive and canola oil -keep saturated and trans-fats to less than 5% of total calories]. About 10 to 15% in high quality protein [minimal animal fat]

APPENDIX B

Recommended foods by nutrient density, glycemic index and fiber

Ranked from top [best] to bottom. - by best combination of

1. Nutrient density
2. Glycemic Index
3. Fiber

VEGETABLES - raw and fresh preferred. Frozen and canned [no salt added] acceptable

Broccoli
Sweet potato
Carrots
Kale
Spinach
Brussels sprouts
Cabbage
Winter squash
Chard
Corn
Cauliflower
Mushrooms

Green peas Hominy
Peas
Romaine lettuce
Endive
Asparagus
Beets
Hechima
Escarole
Celery
Chinese cabbage
Tomato
Eggplant
Shiitake mushrooms
Green beans
Turnip
Green pepper
Lettuce
Potato
Onions
Summer squash
Vegetable juices
Zucchini

LEGUMES

Soybeans
Black beans
Lentils
Kidney beans
Lentils
Lima beans
Pinto beans
Peas, fresh
Peas, split
White beans

WHOLE GRAINS - BEST -

Brown rice
Whole grain breads and rolls
Whole grain Cereals
Whole grain Crackers
Whole grain Pasta
Buckwheat
Barley
Bran, wheat
Bran, oat
Corn tortillas
Granola
Oatmeal
Popcorn [no oil]

Most whole grain or cereal products that are unprocessed or do not have saturated fat, trans-fats [hydrogenated oil] or significant sugars added.

PROCESSED GRAINS - Unbleached and Enriched [processed] - minimize

Bagels
Crackers
English Muffins
Flour noodles and tortillas
French bread
White rice
Pancakes and Waffles
Pasta
White bread, rolls and buns.
White flour

Most grains or cereals that are processed [not whole grain] and have sugars, hydrogenated oil, plus a multitude of other chemicals are simple carbohydrates and should be kept to a minimum.

FRUITS [ranked best from top by blend of most nutrient rich, highest fiber and lowest GI]

Apple
Dates
Blueberries
Blackberries
Raisins
Orange
Banana
Figs
Grapes
Cranberries
Raspberries
Prunes
Kiwifruit
Lemon
Apricot
Grapefruit
Cantaloupe
Plum
Mango
Citrus Juices
Guava
Fruit juices
Honeydew melon
Asian pear
Nectarine
Papaya
Strawberries
Passion fruit
Peach
Pear
Cherries
Tangerine

Persimmons
Pineapple
Plantain
Prickly pear
Rhubarb
Star fruit
Watermelon

CALCIUM RICH FOODS - 2-3 servings a day

Low-fat or fat free dairy products - cheese, yogurt, sour cream yogurt and skim milk
Tofu
Soy milk, calcium fortified
Soy beans
Kale
Optional or rarely - whole milk, ice cream, creams, cheese and any high saturated fat food

FLAVONOID FOODS - 2-4 servings daily

Flaxseed
Soy flakes
Soy concentrate
Soy flour
Soy nuts
Miso
Tofu
Tempeh
Onions
Cranberry juice
Kale
Celery
Broccoli
Soy noodles
Green tea

Soy milk
Chickpeas
Applesauce
Strawberries
Grapes
Green peppers
Lentils
Beans
Lentils

OMEGA-3 FOODS – 1-3 servings daily

Fish ranked high in omega 3 and low in mercury
Atlantic salmon
Sardines
Rainbow trout
Coho salmon, wild
Tuna [canned only]
Flaxseed
Soy products
Soybean oil
Walnuts
Nuts
Beans, Kidney Navy and Soy

GOOD FATS

Canola oil
Flaxseed oil
Olive oil
Peanut oil
Nuts
Soybeans [toasted]

OPTIONAL FATS - occasional

Corn oil

Safflower oil
Soybean oil
Sunflower oil

BAD FATS - Saturated and Trans Fats - avoid as much as possible

Red Meat
Butter
Coconut oil
Dairy fat
Margarine
Palm oil
Animal fat
Most baked goods
Hydrogenated oils
Processed foods with trans-fats [hydrogenated oils]
Pastries, cookies and pies
Many processed foods

NUTS & SEEDS -one serving a day

Almonds
Peanuts
Sunflower seeds
Walnuts
Brazil
Cashews

THERAPEUTIC FOODS AND HERBS - Optional

Turmeric – Widely used in Japan, China and India as a curry spice from the ginger family. It is claimed to have considerable medicinal properties, most importantly is its use as an anti-inflammatory. It is approved for such use by Germany and is considered safe by the FDA. India is has a very high rate of use as it is used in virtually all their foods. Since India has one of the lowest rates of Alzheimer's disease in the world, there are claims that there is a direct association. The best way to consume turmeric is a spice on recommended foods.

APPENDIX C

Typical Menus

Use as guide only, may be interchanged and substituted with similar types of foods.

BREAKFAST	LUNCH	DINNER
Day One		
· 2 toaster whole grain waffles · 2 tbs. Maple syrup · 1/2 cup orange juice · 1 cup tea or coffee **Morning snack** 1/2 cantaloupe 1 cup of green or black tea	· 1 serving Lentil soup-low fat · Green salad · 1 whole fruit **Afternoon snack** 3 oz. Nonfat yogurt	· 3 oz. salmon, broiled with lemon · 1 small yam baked with 1/2 cup nonfat yogurt · 1/2 cups kale with nonfat dressing · 1 serving roasted vegetables
Day Two		
· 1-2 cups whole grain cereal with handful of dried fruit and skim milk · 1 cup coffee or tea **Morning snack** 1/2 oz. of roasted nuts	· Chinese tomato salad · 1 baked potato with marinara sauce · 3 whole grain crackers **Afternoon snack** Raw carrot	* Chicken Curry 1 serving · 1/2 cup steamed asparagus · 1/2 cup wild rice · fruit cup

Day Three		
· 1 poached egg · 1 slice whole-wheat bread · 1/2 grapefruit **Morning snack** · 1 pcs raw vegetable	· Veggie sandwich of · 2 slices whole grain bread with 1 slice of low fat cheese, 2 leaves of romaine lettuce and 2 slices of tomato with a dash of olive oil. · 1 cup tea · **Afternoon snack** 1 fresh whole fruit	· 1 serving Sweet and Sour Pork · Spinach with sesame seeds · 1 whole grain roll · nonfat yogurt with fruit topping
Week one - Day Four		
· 1 cup of low fat whole grain cereal · 1 sliced banana · skim milk · 1 cup coffee **Morning snack** 1 pcs of whole fruit	3 cups Green salad with nonfat dressing · 3 whole wheat crackers · 1 sm. baked sweet potato **Afternoon snack** · 1 cup tea · 4 grape tomatoes	· Moroccan Vegetable Stew - 1 serving · 1/2 cup Couscous · Greek salad * Fresh berries with 1/2 cup of nonfat yogurt
Week One - Day Five		
· Whole grain bagel with 2 tbs. peanut butter · 6 whole, pitted dates · 1 cup coffee **Morning snack** 1/2 oz. of sunflower seeds	· Salmon sandwich with 3 oz. canned salmon, on 2 slices of whole-wheat bread, with 2 leaves of lettuce, 1 slice of onion and 2 slices of tomato · 6-8 oz. skim milk · Afternoon snack · 1 pc whole fruit	Vegetables a la Grecque* · 1 baked potato with · nonfat dressing · 1 whole grain roll · mixed fruit cup
Week One - Day Six		
· Grapefruit broiled with dash of brown sugar · 2 oz. of egg whites or egg substitute with chopped onion and sweet pepper · 1 slice whole grain toast	· 2 cups Spinach/mush-room · salad with chopped sweet peppers and lemon juice · 1 whole wheat roll **Afternoon Snack** 1 cup of tea 1/3 cup roasted soy beans	· Baked Mackerel "Plaki" style* - 2 oz. · Greek salad · 1 med baked potato · 1/3 cup rizogalo · 6 oz. nonfat yogurt with fruit topping

Week One Day seven		
· 2 -5inch Whole wheat pancakes with dash of olive oil, one egg white and soy beverage · Topped with blueberries · Cup of orange juice · Cup of coffee	· One cup whole wheat pasta with olive oil and topped with 1 tbs. Parmesan cheese and parsley · Green salad with tomatoes with no fat salad dressing **Afternoon snack** * 10 whole almonds	· Sicilian Stuffed Peppers 1- serving · 1/2 cup whole grain pasta with dash of Olive oil and chopped tomatoes · 2 multi-grain rolls with nonfat spread 1/4 cup of low fat ice cream with berries.
Week Two - Day One	**Restaurant**	
· 1 cup of low fat whole grain cereal · 1 sliced banana · skim milk · 1 cup coffee **Morning snack** 1 pc of whole fruit	· 1 cup Whole wheat spaghetti with marinara sauce · 1/2 cup steamed eggplant · Green salad **Afternoon snack** · 1/2 cup grapes	· Chinese Cabbage rolls with tofu and chicken - 1 serving · 1 whole grain roll · 1/2 cup low fat ice cream with fruit topping.
Week Two - Day Two	**Restaurant**	
· Omelet -1 serving with eggbeaters, chopped sweet peppers and onion. stir fried with olive oil. · 1 slice toasted whole grain rye bread · 6-8 oz. orange juice · cup coffee or tea **Morning snack** · 1 pcs fruit	· 2 cups salad bar with low · fat dressing · Baked potato with dash of fat free dressing. **Afternoon snack** · 1/2 whole wheat pita with 1 tsp. of low fat peanut butter · 1 cup tea	· Fettuccine Alfredo 1 serving · Green salad with olive oil vingerette · 1 rye whole grain roll · 1/2 cup of nonfat yogurt with cherries
Week Two - Day Three		
· 1/2 cantaloupe · 1/3 cup blueberries · 1 slice whole grain bread · 1 egg white fried in Olive oil · 1 glass orange juice **Morning snack** · 1 oz. seeds	· Black-Bean Soup - 1 serving · Green salad · 3 whole grain crackers **Afternoon snack** · 1 cup unsalted vegetable juice	· Steamed Vegetables with 1/3 cup cauliflower, 1/2 cup broccoli, 1 sliced carrot, 1/4 cup kale, 1/2 cup green string beans topped with nonfat Italian dressing. · fruit cup

Week Two - Day Four	Chinese Restaurant	

· 1-2 Cups whole grain
· cereal, dried fruit and
  1/2 oz. nuts
· 1/2 cup soy milk
· 1/2 cup skim milk
Morning snack
· 1 pcs raw vegetable
	· Steamed vegetables
	  with
	· minimum soy sauce-1
	  serving
	· 1/3 cup rice
	Afternoon snack
	1 pc whole fruit
		· Tempeh Burger on
		· mixed grain bun, with 1
		  tsp. Tomato paste, 1 tsp
		  mustard 1 slice onion
		  and romaine leaves
		· Banana Milkshake with
		  1 cup skim milk and 1
		  banana whipped

Week Two - Day Five		**Restaurant**

· 3/4 cup 1 min. Oat-
  meal
· 1/2 cup soy/skim milk
· 1/4 cup raisins
· 1 cup coffee
Morning snack
· 1 oz. seeds
	· cup low fat canned
	  minestrone soup
	· Green salad
	· 3 whole grain crackers
	Afternoon snack
	· cup applesauce
		· 3 oz. Filet of sole,
		  broiled with lemon and
		  herbs
		· 1/2 cup steamed car-
		  rots
		· 2 cups tossed green
		  salad with nonfat dress-
		  ing
		· 21md baked potato
		  with no fat dressing
		· 1/2 cup fresh fruit

Week Two - Day Six		

· Banana bread with
  olive oil and 1/2 oz.
  sunflower seeds made
  with whole grain flour
· 1 fresh orange
· 1 cup green or black
  tea
Morning snack
· 1 cup tea
· 1 oz. nuts
	· 2 cups Chief salad
	  with oz. fresh turkey,
	  and assorted fresh
	  vegetables and fat free
	  dressing
	· 4 rye crackers, unsalted
	Afternoon snack
	· whole grain bagel with
	  tsp. fruit jam
		· Chinese Bai Zai
		  Chicken
		· Vegetable rice with
		  walnuts
		· 1/2 cup vegetarian
		  baked beans
		· Pear-Lemon-Ginger
		  Shake

Week Two - Day Seven		

· 1/2 cantaloupe
· 1/3 cup blueberries
· 1/4 cup of eggbeaters
· 1 slice whole grain
  bread - toasted
· 1 cup skim milk
Morning snack
· 1 cup tea
· 1 oz. seeds
	· 1 cup Tuna salad - 1
	  serving
	· whole wheat pita
	Afternoon snack
	 cup nonfat yogurt with
	 fruit toppling.
		· Italian Country Lin-
		  guine
		· 1/2 cup brussel
		  sprouts
		· 1-whole grain roll
		· 1/2 cup canned mixed
		  fruit

Week Three - Day One		
· 2 toaster whole grain · waffles · 2 tbs. Maple syrup · 1/2 cup orange juice · 1 cup tea or coffee **Morning snack** Low calorie snack 1 cup of green or black tea	· Black-Bean Soup - 1 serving · Green salad * · 3 whole grain crackers **Afternoon snack** · 1 cup unsalted vegetable juice	· Mu Shu Chicken - 1 serving · 1/2 cup curried vegetable and tofu soup · 1 med baked yam · 1 fruit cup
Week Three - Day Two		
· 1 cup of low fat whole grain cereal · 1 sliced banana · skim milk · 1 cup coffee **Morning snack** 1 pcs of whole fruit	3 cups Green salad with nonfat dressing · 3 whole wheat crackers · 1 sm. baked sweet potato · Afternoon snack · 1 cup tea · 1 tsp. low fat peanut butter on cracker	· Vegetables and Salmon · 1 lb. Mixed frozen vegetables, cooked · 1-1/4 cups mushrooms, sliced and cooked · 1/3 can pink salmon, water packed 1/2 cup pasta sauce
Week Three - Day Three		
· Omelet with following · 1/2 cup eggbeaters or 2 egg whites · 1/4 cup chopped sweet red peppers · 1/4 cup chopped onions · 1 slice toasted whole grain bread **Morning snack** 6-8 oz. orange juice	· Salmon sandwich with 3 oz. canned salmon, on 2 slices of whole-wheat bread, with 2 leaves of lettuce, 1 slice of onion and 2 slices of tomato · 6-8 oz. skim milk **Afternoon snack** · 1 pcs whole fruit	· 2 oz. turkey breast, deli or roasted, no skin on whole grain bread · 1/2 baked sweet potato · 1 large broccoli spear, steamed · Green salad, any combo with 2 tbsp. fat free salad dressing
Week Three - Day Four		
· instant oatmeal with 3/4 cup of instant oatmeal, 1 cup of soy/skim milk* · Topped with 1 sliced banana	· Spinach/mushroom · Salad - 2 cups · with chopped sweet peppers and lemon juice · 1 whole wheat roll **Afternoon Snack** 1 cup tea 1/3 cup roasted soy beans	· 3 oz. pink salmon, broiled · with 3/4 cup tomato sauce · 1 med. sweet potato, baked · 1 cup peas and onions[frozen, prepared] · 6 oz. nonfat yogurt with fruit topping

Week Three - Day Five		
· 1 serving scrambled Tofu* · 1 slice mixed-grain bread · 1/2 grapefruit · 1 cup tea or coffee **Morning snack** · 1/2 grapefruit · 1 cup tea	· 1 serving Lentil soup- low fat · Green salad* · 1 whole fruit · **Afternoon snack** · cup tea · 2 oz. nuts	· Pasta Primavera - 1 serving · 1/3 cup lima beans · 1/2 cup stewed toma- toes · 1 whole grain roll · mixed fruit
Week Three - Day Six	**Chinese restaurant**	
· 1-1/4 cups rolled oats, cooked with · 1/4 cup wheat bran · 1 sliced banana · 1 glass skim milk	· Steamed vegetables with · minimum soy sauce-1 · serving · 1/3 cup rice **Afternoon snack** 1 pc whole fruit	· Baked Mackerel "Plaki" · Style* - 1 serving · Greek salad · 1 med. baked potato · 1/3 cup rizogalo
Week Three - Day Seven		
· 1 cup of low fat whole grain cereal · 1 sliced banana · 1/2 cup skim milk · 1 cup coffee **Morning snack** 1 pcs of whole fruit	· **1 cup**-Tuna salad* · whole wheat pita · 1 cup tea **Afternoon snack** cup nonfat yogurt with fruit toppling.	· Cranberry-Glazed Chicken Breast with whole grain stuffing* 1 serving · 1/2 Brussels sprouts · 1/2 cup carrot salad · 1/2 cup frozen fat free yogurt
Week Four - Day One		
· Omelet* with eggbeat- ers, chopped sweet peppers and onion. stir fried with olive oil. · 1 slice toasted whole grain rye bread · 6-8 oz. orange juice · cup coffee or tea	· 1 serving Lentil soup- low fat · Green salad* · 1 whole fruit **Afternoon snack** 2 oz. nuts 1 cup tea	· Baked Mackerel "Plaki" · Style* 1-serving. · Greek salad* · 1 med. baked potato · 1/3 cup rizogalo · fruit cup
Week Four - Day Two		
· 1/2 cup low fat Gra- nola · 1/4 cup berries · 1/2 cup soy/skim milk **Morning snack** · 1 cup assoc. raw veg- etables	· **1 cup**-Tuna salad · whole wheat pita **Afternoon snack** cup nonfat yogurt with fruit toppling.	· Japanese simmered soybeans*- 1 serving · Simmered acorn squash* · 1/3 cup wild rice · 3 kumquats with sauce · 1 cup green tea

Week Four - Day Three		

· 1-2 Cups whole grain
· cereal, dried fruit and
  1/2 oz. nuts
· 1/2 cup soy beverage
· 1/2 cup skim milk
Morning snack
· 1 cup tea
· low fat snack
	· Veggie sandwich
	· 2 slices whole grain
	  bread with 1 slice of low
	  fat cheese, 2 leaves of
	  romaine lettuce and 2
	  slices of tomato with a
	  dash of olive oil
	Morning snack
	· 1 fresh whole fruit
		· Beef and Green bean
		  stir fry* - 1 serving
		· Green Salad*
		· 1 whole grain roll
		· mixed fruit

Week Four - Day Four		

1-1/4 cups rolled oats,
cooked with 1/4 cup
wheat bran
1 sliced banana
1 glass skim milk
	· Pita-bread pizza*1-serv.
	· Cup of minestrone
	  soup
	Afternoon snack
	· 1/2 cup cherry toma-
	  toes
		· 2-3 oz. Broiled halibut
		· Steamed artichoke
		· 1 med. baked potato
		· 2 cups Salad, Belgian
		  endive, asparagus, yel-
		  low pepper
		· 1/4 cup of berries

Week Four - Day Five	**Fast food restaurant**	

· 1 cup whole wheat
  flakes
· 1/2 cup soy/skim milk
· Sliced banana
Morning snack
· 1/2 fresh orange
	· Veggie sub on wheat
	  bun
	· 1 cup of raw vegetables
	  with sprinkle of olive
	  oil and vinegar
	Afternoon snack
	· 6 oz. unsalted tomato
	  juice
		· Chicken stuffed cab-
		  bage, Japanese style* 1
		  serving
		· 1/2 cup mixed rice
		· 1/2 cup egg drop soup
		· 3 kumquats in sauce

Week Four - Day Six	**Mexican Restaurant**	

· 1/2 cup low fat Gra-
  nola
· 1/4 cup berries
· 1/2 cup soy/skim milk
Morning snack
· 1 cup assoc. raw veg-
  etables
	· 1 soft chicken taco;
	  steamed corn tortilla,
	  chicken, vegetables,
	  salsa
	Afternoon snack
	· 1/3 cup roasted soy
	  beans
		· Poached salmon with
		  dill sauce*
		· Steamed Italian squash
		  and carrots
		· Brown rice
		· 1/2 cup Nonfat ice
		  cream with berries

Week Four - Day Seven		

· OGD omelet [ ] with eggbeaters, chopped sweet peppers and onion. stir fried with olive oil. · 1 slice toasted whole grain rye bread · 6-8 oz. orange juice · cup coffee or tea	· Chinese tomato salad* · 1 baked potato with marinara sauce · 3 whole grain crackers **Afternoon snack** Raw carrot	· Tofu sandwich on whole grain bread with shrimp filling - 1 serving · Miso soup with pork and vegetables*-1 serving · Green salad · 1 rice fortune cookie [opt]

MENU notes

1. Foods with [*] refer to recipe in appendix
2. Foods that do not have quantities can be consumed to satisfaction.
3. Any Breakfast, Lunch or Dinner can be interchanged
4. Convenient meals are listed [mostly for breakfast and lunch] when preparation time may not be available.
5. Grains and Cereals - maximize whole grains and select from recommend list
6. 4-8 oz. of red wine daily [optional]
7. Tea - 1-3 cups of green or black tea daily
8. Coffee - limit to 2 cups daily - nonfat dairy
9. Dressings -All dressings without recipes are available at supermarket in fat-free types
10. Fruits - Select fruits, fresh preferred frozen or canned acceptable, from recommended list and consume a variety.
11. Olive oil - 1-2 tbl spoons daily.

APPENDIX D

List of sources and citations

Chapter 1 -What this book can do for you

Ames, B. Oxidants, antioxidants, and the degenerative diseases of aging. *Proceedings of the National Academy of Sciences* 1993;90[17]:7915-22

Carper, J. Stop Aging Now.. New York: *HarperCollins* 1995

Harman, D. Extending functional life span *Exp Gerontol* 1998 Jan-Mar; 33[1-2]:95-112

Harman,D. Aging, Prospects for increases in the functional life span Age 1994: 17;119-46

Harman,D. The aging process: Major risk factor for disease and death. *Proceedings of the National Academy of Sciences* 1991; 88:5360-63

Harman,D. Aging:Prospects for further increases in the functional life span. *Age* 1994; 17:119-46

National Institute on Aging. *Research on Older Women: Highlights from the Baltimore Longitudinal Study of Aging,* Bethesda, MD: National Institutes of Health, 1991.

Ornish, D. Dr. Dean Ornish's Program for Reversing Heart Disease 1990. Ballantine Books, NY

Perls, Living to 100

Rowe, J & Kahn,R. 1998 <u>Successful Aging.</u> *MacArthur Foundation Study.* Dell Publishing, NY

World Cancer Research Fund, American Institute for Cancer Research. <u>Food, Nutrition and the Prevention of Cancer: a global perspective.</u> Washington, DC.: American Institute for Cancer Research, 1997

Chapter 2 -Genesis of our Obesity Epidemic

Acheson KJ Schutz Y. et al. Glycogen Storage Capacity and De Novo Lipogenesis during Massive Carbohydrate overfeeding in Man. American Journal of Clinical Nutrition. 1988 August, 48(2):2407

Allen, J, Cheer, S. *Civilization and the Thrift Genotype.* Asia Pacific Journal of Clinical Nutrition 4[4] [1995]: 341-342

Branson, R. Horber, F. Kral, J. Hoehe, M. et al: *Binge Eating as a Major Phenotype of Melanocortin 4 Receptor Gene Mutations.* NEJM Vol. 348:1096-1103 20 Mar 03

Chen, J. Campbell, T. Li, J, Petr,R. *Diet, Life-Style and Mortality in China. A study of the Characteristics of 65 Chinese Counties,* Ithaca, NY. Cornell University Press 1990

Eaton SB, Shostak M, Konner M 1998. *The Paleolithic Prescription.* NY, Harper and Row

Food and Agriculture Organization of the United Nations. *Protein quality evaluation* [FAO food and nutrition paper 51] Rome FAO 1990

Garn, S. *From the Miocene to Olestra: An Historical Perspective on Fat Consumption.* Journal of the American Dietetic Association 97 [7] Suppl [July 1997] S54-7

Hamm, P, Shekelle, R and Stamler, J. *Large fluctuations in body weight during your adulthood and the twenty five year risked of coronary disease in men.* Amer J Epidemiology 129[1989" 312-318

Hulas, J., Gavial, K, Mafia, M ET all *"Weight Reducing Effects in the Plasma Protein Encoded by the obese Gene.* Science 269 [1995]: 543-546

Journal of the American Medical Association *Portion sizes, etc.* JAMA Jan22/29 2003

Journal of the American Dietetic Association *Portion sizes on certain foods from 1990 to 1995.* JADA. Jan 2003

Keesey, R. *A Set Point Theory of Obesity. In* Brownell a, K and Forety, H. *Handbook of Eating Disorders: Physiology, Psychology and Treatment of Obesity.* New York, Basic Books, 1986. 63-87

Manson, J, Willett, W, et al. *Body Weight and Mortality among Women.* New England Journal of Medicine 333[11] [September 15, 1995] 677-685

Montague, C, Farooqi, Il et al. *Congenital Leftin Deficiency is Associated with Severe Early Onset Obesity in Humans.* Nature 387 [June 26 1997]

Manson, J, Willett, W, et al. *Body Weight ad Mortality among Women.* New England Journal of Medicine 333[11] [September 15, 1995] 677-685

Nielsen, S. Popkin, B. *Patterns and Trends in Food Portion Sizes, 1977-1998.* The Journal of the American Medical Association [JAMA] Vp;/289 No. 4, Jan 22 2003

Nielsen, SJ, Popkin BM, et al. *'Trends in Energy Intake in U.S. between 1977 and 1996* Obesity Research 10:370-378 [2002]

Schlosser, E, *Fast Food Nation: The Dark Side of the All-American Meal.* Boston: Houghton Mifflin, 2001

Shell, E. *The Hungry Gene, The science of Fat and the Future of Thin.* N.Y Atlantic Monthly Press 2002

Stearns, P. *Fat History Bodies and Beauty in the Modern West* New York. New York University Press, 1997

World Cancer Research Fund/American Institute for Cancer Research. *Food, Nutrition the Prevention of Cancer: a Global Perspective 1997* American Institute for Cancer Research

Chapter 3 - Why weight loss program can be weight gain programs

Atkins C: *Dr. Atkins' New Diet Revolution* NY. Avon Books; 1999

Drenick EJ, Brickman AS, et al. *Dissociation of the obesity-hyperinsulin-ism relationship Following dietary restriction and hyperalimentation.* Am J Clin Nutr. 1972;25746-755

Eades MR, Eades MD. *Protein Power.* NY ; Bantam Books 1996

Freedman MR. *Popular Diets: A Scientific Review.* Washington, DC: USDA Office of Research, Education and Economics; 2001:1-8

Holt SH. Brand-Miller JC. Et al. Satiety Index of Common Foods. European Journal of Clinical Nutrition, 1995; 49:675-690

Kennedy, ET, Bowman, SA, et al. *Popular diets; correlation to health, nutrition, and obesity.* J. Am Diet Assoc. 2001;101:411-420

Klem ML, Wing RR, et al A Descriptive Study of Individuals Successful at Long- term Maintenance of Substantial Weight Loss American Journal of Clinical Nutrition 1997;66:239-246

Larosa JC Gry AG, et al. Effects of high-protein. *Low carbohydrate dieting on plasma lipoproteins and body weight* J. Am Diet Assoc. 1980;264-270 Academy Press 1989. Lipids. Pp44-51

D.C.; Pritikin National Research Council. Recommended Dietary Allowances. Washing, National RP 'The Pritikin Weight Loss Breakthrough' 1998 NY Penguin Putnam Inc.

Sears B. *The Zone.* NY: Harper Collins; 1995

Serdula MK, Mokdad AH, Williamson DF, et al. Prevalence of attempting weight loss and strategies for controlling weight JAMA 1999;282:1353-1358].

Stillman IM Baker SS. *The Doctor's Quick Weight Loss Diet,* NY: Dell Publishing; 1967

Tremblay A. Nutritional determinants of he insulin resistance syndrome Int J Obes Relat Metab Disord 1995;[suppl 1] S60-S68

Yost TJ, Jensen DR, et al. Effect of dietary macronutrient composition on tissue- specific lipoprotein lipase activity and Insuli9n action in normal-weight subjects. Am J Clin Nutr. 1998;68:296-302

Chapter 4 –The worlds healthiest and longest lived peoples

Campbell TC. Junshi C. Diet and Chronic; Degenerative Diseases; Perspective from China American Journal of Clinical Nutrition. 1994 May, 59(5 Suppl); 1153S- 1161S.

Cambell, C, Cambell, T. The China Study: The Most Comprehensive Study of Nutrition Ever Conducted and the Startling Implications for Diet, Weight Loss and Long-Term Health. BenBella Books, Dallas TX [2004]

Keys A. Seven Countries: A Multivariate Analysis of Death and Coronary Heart Disease Commonwealth Fund Publications) [1980]

Keys A. How to eat well and stay well the Mediterranean way DoubleDay [1975]

Willcox B, Willcox D, Suzuki M. The Okinawa Program – How the World's longest- lived people achieve everlasting health-and how you can too. Clarkson Potter Publisher NY[2001]

World Health Organization. Epidemiology and Prevention of Cardiovascular Diseases in Elderly People. WHO Technical Report Series 853. Geneva

Chapter 5 – The OGD eating program

American Heart Association Science Advisory, entitled Dietary Protein and Weight Reduction, by Sachiko T. St. Jeor, ED, Howard, BV, et al and published in 'Circulation. 2001;104: 1869-1874,

Flatt JP. Use and Storage of Carbohydrate and Fat. American Journal of Clinical Nutrition's 1995 April, 61 (4 Suppl) 952S-959S

Foster, G. Wyatt, H. Hill J. et al. *A Randomized Trial of a Low-Carbohydrate Diet for Obesity.* NEJM Vol 348:2082-2090, Num 21, May 22 2003

Haber G. Depletion and Disruption of Dietary Fiber. Effects on Satiety, Plasma-Glucose and Serum-Insulin. Lancet. 1977;2:679

Hass, E. M. Staying Healthy with Nutrition

Jenkins DJ Jenkins AL. Et al. Low Glycemic Index: Lente Carbohydrates and Physiological Effects of Altered Food Frequency. American Journal of Clinical Nutrition. 1994,59-706S-709S

Kendall A. Levitsky DA, et al. Weight Loss on a Low-fat Diet: Consequence on the Imprecision of the Control of Food Intake in

Humans. American Journal Clinical Nutrition. 1991;53:1124-1129

Lissner, L. Levitsky, DA et al Dietary Fat and the Regulation of Energy Intake I Human Subjects. American Journal of Clinical Nutrition, 1987,46:886-892.

Mates RD Fat Preference and Adherence to a Reduced -fat Diet, American Journal of Clinical Nutrition, 1993, 57(3); 373-81

NIH Technology Assessment Conference Panel. Methods for Voluntary Weight Loss and Control. Annals of Internal Medicine. 1993;119;764-770

Rowe, J & Kahn,R. 1998 Successful Aging. *MacArthur Foundation study*. Dell Publishing,

Rusting, R. Why do we age? *Scientific American* 1992;267 [6]:130

Walford, R. The clinical promise of diet restriction. *Geriatrics* 1990;45[4]: 81-83,86-87

Weindruch, R., and Walford, R.L., *The Retardation of Aging and Disease by Dietary Restriction,* Springfield, IL: Charles C. Thomas, 1988.

Chapter 6-How the EMP behavioral program makes it work

Benson, H. The Relaxation Response. A study of the biological effects of human response to meditation.

Borysenko, J & Morysenko, M. The power of the Mind to Heal. 1995 Carlsbad, CA Hay House.

Dossey, L. Healing Words; The Power of Prayer and the Practice of Medicine. San Francisco; HarperCollins. 1995

Goldman, D, Gurin, J. Mind Body Medicine; How to Use your Mind for Better Health. Yonkers, NY. Consumer Reports Books

Henderson, C. Self Hypnosis for the life you want 2003. New York, New York

Kabat-Zinn, J. Wherever You Go There You Are : mindfulness meditation in everyday life. 1994. New York, Hyperion

Kabat-Zinn, J. Full Catastrophe Living; Using the Wisdom of Your Body and Mind to Face Stress, Pain and Illness. 1990 New York: Delta

Kabat-Zinn, J, et al 1985. The clinical use of mindfulness meditation for the self- regulation of chronic pain. J. Behav. Med. 8:163:190

Kabat-Zinn, J, et al 1986. Four-year follow-up of meditation-based program for the self- regulation of chronic pain. Clin. J. Pain 2:150-173

LeCron, L. The Complete Guide to Hypnosis 1971 New York, Harper & Row

National Institutes of Health Alternative Medicine" expanding medical horizons. NIH Publication No. 94-066, Dec 1994

Rossman,M, 2000. Guided imagery for self-healing: an essential resource for anyone seeking wellness. Tiburon, CA. H.J. Kramer

Thich Nhat Hanh. 1975. The Miracle of Mindfulness.N.Y. Riverhead Books

Weil, A. Spontaneous Healing: How to Discover and Enhance Your Body's Natural Ability to Maintain and Heal Itself. NY: Ballantine Books 1996

Chapter 7 -Physical Activity

Coyle EF. Substrate Utilization during Exercise in Active People. American Journal of Clinical Nutrition. 1995 April, 61(4 Suppl);968S-979S

Fiatarone, M.A., Marks, E.C., et al., "High-IntensityStrength Training in Nonagenarians," *Journals of the American Medical Association*1990 263:3029-3034,

Gilbert, S., Editor. Improving Memory. Understand and Preventing Age-Related Memory Loss. Harvard Health Pub. Boston MA

Jakicic, J, Marcus, B. et al. Effect of Exercise Duration and Intensity on Weight Loss in Overweight, Sedentary Women JAMA 2003; 290: 1323-1330

Mayo Clinic Health Letter. *Managing your* Weight', Feb 2003.

McArdle WD. Katch FL Essentials of Exercise Physiology, Philadelphia; Lea & Febiger, 1994 Rolls BJ Carbohydrates, Fats, and Satiety American Journal of Clinical Nutrition, 1995 April, 61 Supplement 4:960S-967S

NIH Publication No 96 4031, April 1996. E-text by NIDDK posted 20 Feb. 1998

Schuit, et al. National Institute of Pubic Health, the described in *Medicine & Science in Sports & Exercise* 2001;33:772-777 and reported in Reuters Health information Wed, May 2, 2001.

Sherman, S.E. et al. Comparison of past verses recent physical activity I the prevention of premature death and coronary artery disease *Am Heart J.* 1999;138:90- 907

Weil, A. Strength Training for Everyone. Jan 2001. *Self Healing.* Thorne Communications, Watertown, MA

Zachwiega JJ. Exercise as Treatment for Obesity. Endocrinology and Metabolism Clinics of North American . 1996 December

END

SUBMISSION CHECKLIST

Customer Profile

James D. Baird PhD
934 Cherry Hills Lane
Naperville, IL 60563
630 420 2311
drjamesdbaird@aol.com

Author Biography

James D. Baird, PhD, was an inventor-engineer for over 30 years and after retiring, acquired a PhD in Natural Health to further his personal interests of genetics and health. Baird was amazed at the lack of success with diets and after researching the subject, wrote *Obesity Genes and how to turn them off with epigenetic modifiers*

Endorsements

Dr. Baird has succeeded where others have failed. He has identified the genetic and unhealthy eating habits that cause overweight and obesity, and provided solutions. The proven diets of the world's healthiest people are adopted with new eating habits facilitated by special epigenetic programs that can turn off our Obesity Genes.

Brenda Madura RN,BSN,MS,CNM

Dr Baird has pinpointed the causes of failure to maintain diets, and in so doing, is able to provide practical ways that busy people can permanently change their eating behavior. I hope to use it in my medical practice.

Edward R. Rosick, DO, MPH,

Reading Line

Diets don't work because they fail to modify our obesity genes. The new science of epigenetics provides the means to do that

Bullet Points

- Overweight is due to our Obesity Genes
- The Genesis of our obesity epidemic
- The Worlds healthiest and longest lived [HALL] peoples
- The Obesity Gene eating program
- Taming our Obesity Genes with Epigenetics

Book Description

Obesity Genes uncovers the reasons why diets don't work.- ancient genetic food drives and unhealthy eating habits. The genes that permitted our ancestors to survive, during the period when calories were scarce, motivated them to prefer high calorie fats, sweets and more calories. These same 'obesity' genes are out of sync with present day needs, but still drive our food preferences.

The Obesity Genes Diet acknowledges our urges and satisfies our genes with healthy types of fat, sweets, and calories. It adopts the diet of the world's longest living and healthiest peoples, by blending the best and tastiest foods from the Mediterranean, Asian and Okinawa diets. However, it is unrealistic to think that our unhealthy eating habits, encouraged by the availability of high calorie foods, can be changed by will power.

Because we are creatures of habit and food preference is learned, the only successful way to a long term diet is to develop healthy eating habits. To meet this requirement, the book provides a step by step program of epigenetic interventions directed at modifying our obesity genes and developing healthy eating habits. These interventions include; mindful eating, relaxation response, self-hypnosis and self-guided imagery. The key to facilitating these interventions is to develop more consciousness by understanding how the mind works.

Copyright holder
James D. Baird 2012